Henrietta Norton is a nutritional therapist who specialises in fertility and pregnancy. She has a clinic at the integrated medical practice Grace Belgravia alongside the apothecary to HM The Queen Dr Tim Evans. She is a member of the British Association of Nutritional Therapists (BANT) and an associate member of the Royal Society of Medicine and the Guild of Health Writers. She is also a foresight preconception practitioner, functional medicine AFMCP graduate and is currently completing her MSc in nutritional medicine at the University of Surrey. Henrietta is co-founder of food supplement brand Wild Nutrition and the author of *Take Control of Your Endometriosis*.

In addition, Henrietta is a mother to three young children and understands the trials and tribulations of pregnancy and birth first-hand.

YOUR
PREGNANCY
NUTRITION
GUIDE

WHAT TO EAT WHEN YOU'RE PREGNANT

HENRIETTA NORTON

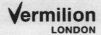

Vermilion
LONDON

3 5 7 9 10 8 6 4 2

Vermilion, an imprint of Ebury Publishing,
20 Vauxhall Bridge Road,
London SW1V 2SA

Vermilion is part of the Penguin Random House group of companies
whose addresses can be found at global.penguinrandomhouse.com

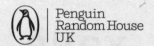

Copyright © Henrietta Norton 2015

Henrietta Norton has asserted her right to be identified as the author of this
Work in accordance with the Copyright, Designs and Patents Act 1988

First published by Vermilion in 2015

www.eburypublishing.co.uk

A CIP catalogue record for this book is available from the British Library

ISBN 9780091955168

Penguin Random House is committed to a sustainable future for
our business, our readers and our planet. This book is made from
Forest Stewardship Council® certified paper.

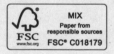

Printed and bound in Great Britain by Clays Ltd, St Ives plc

CONTENTS

To Alfie, Ned and Oscar Norton.

I love you deeply, for all that you are and will become.

INTRODUCTION

'Gardeners know that you must nourish the soil if
you want healthy plants. You must water the plants
adequately, especially when seeds are germinating and
sprouting, and they should be planted in a nutrient-rich
soil. Why should nutrition matter less in the creation
of young humans than it does in young plants?'

Ina May Gaskin, *Ina May's Guide to Childbirth*

You are likely to have picked up this book because you have already entered the nine months transition to motherhood. You have started on the journey that many women have travelled before you and many will do so after you. Pregnancy is a wonderful act of nature and a miraculous time – you and your baby have become part of the natural cycle of life. Whether you are four weeks or four months pregnant, your nurturing relationship with your baby has already begun.

In this book, I offer you advice and information on the valuable nutritional changes that can make you and your growing baby healthier. As a nutritional therapist, I am fortunate to work with many women during an important and treasured time in their lives, from the preconception period (whether supporting fertility treatment or natural fertility) through to pregnancy and the early stages of motherhood. This work, as well as my scientific research on nutrition during pregnancy, compound my passionate belief that good nutrition has a vital role to play in the health and development of the unborn child.

SOUND ADVICE

There is so much conflicting information about what is safe during pregnancy: how much caffeine or alcohol you can have, how to reduce the risk of allergies in your baby, and whether or not you should be taking supplements. This book is not about focusing on what you 'can't have' or scaremongering about getting everything right. It's about providing truly helpful expert information, which is clear rather than confusing, based on the latest research on nutrition during pregnancy. My aim is to support you and offer sound advice and wisdom that I have drawn on from my experience as a nutritional therapist specialising in fertility and pregnancy, as well as a mother of three myself.

Pregnancy is an emotional and spiritual experience, as well as a physical one. Your mental well-being and how to emotionally prepare for the transition from pregnant woman to new mother is discussed throughout the book too.

YOUR QUESTIONS ANSWERED

I will show you how easy it is to eat a healthy diet every day. I will answer the all-important questions, such as which foods to eat and which foods to avoid during pregnancy; the important nutrients for each trimester and in which foods to find them; how good nutrition can support symptoms such as morning sickness, and how it can help you prepare for birth and breastfeeding. I'll look at blood-sugar levels and the best way to maintain them, how to supplement your diet with extra vitamins, and how to keep your energy levels up during those exhausting few months after giving birth.

I know that, despite our best intentions, it is not always easy to eat in the most nourishing way. I want to show you how you can make small changes to your diet that can transform your health. By using delicious recipes to do so (see Chapter 14), these changes will feel exciting – and the food you'll be eating will taste great! I'll also give you lots of practical strategies, such as a store-cupboard shopping list and menu plans, to make sure that you always have something nourishing to hand. You can use the downloadable 'foods to avoid' list to make food shopping or eating out simple, and the 'pregnancy superfoods' list as a reminder of the hero foods to look for www.henriettanorton.com/about/books.

Each pregnancy is different and so the suggestions made in this book are not strict guidelines. They are simply an aid to empower you to make choices that you feel are right for the well-being of you and your child.

HOW TO USE THIS BOOK

I've designed this book so it's an easy-to-use, handy reference guide for you to dip into over the next few months. There is no need to read it cover to cover in one sitting; instead you may want to take each chapter as you need to, depending on your thirst for information or your stage of pregnancy.

CHAPTERS AT A GLANCE

Chapter 1: Discover the simple changes that you can make to support your pregnancy even before you conceive, including foods to boost, those to reduce, and the effects of lifestyle influences such as stress and caffeine.

Chapter 2: Understand why you and your baby are what you eat, and how your food choices and eating patterns during pregnancy can lay the foundations of good health for both of you. In this chapter, I have summarised the latest research on nutrition and development, and the short- and long-term implications for your health and that of your unborn baby.

Chapter 3: Learn the fundamentals of a healthy diet during pregnancy, and why maintaining a healthy blood-sugar level is so important during pregnancy and early motherhood. We will look at simple ways to maximise your nutrient intake through the way you shop for your food and how you cook it.

Chapter 4: Discover why it is key to good health to get the right balance of macronutrients – fats, protein and carbohydrates. I will answer common questions, such as 'Should I choose margarine over butter?' and 'Should I limit my intake of red meat?'

Chapter 5: Find out why specific vitamins and minerals, known as micronutrients, are needed to support the healthy growth of your baby. Using a why, where and how system, you will learn why you need them, where you can find them and how much you need.

Chapter 6: Familiarise yourself with the complete checklist of foods you need to avoid during pregnancy, including suggestions for helpful substitutes to replace these foods. Also discover how to prepare and store food safely, and how to read nutrition labels.

Chapter 7: A healthy diet is without doubt the most important way to obtain essential nutrients. However, before, during and after pregnancy, there is clear evidence that certain supplements are beneficial. Here I draw on the expertise I have gathered over the years on taking supplements,

Chapter 8: Eating well when you're a vegetarian or vegan can be more of a challenge during pregnancy. In this chapter, discover how to eat well and avoid the common pitfalls of a vegetarian or vegan diet during pregnancy. Learn how to plan your dietary choices to ensure you have the right balance of protein and important nutrients such as iron, vitamin B12 and zinc.

Chapter 9: Not many pregnant women escape the ensuing nine months without experiencing a bout of morning sickness or insomnia, but there are many foods that can help to reduce these symptoms. This chapter offers natural solutions for common pregnancy symptoms including morning sickness, cramps, cravings and constipation.

Chapter 10: Diet can play a significantly supportive role in the body's ability to prepare for labour. Find out how to build your nutrient stores in the last few weeks of pregnancy and prepare your body and your kitchen cupboards for the arrival of your baby.

Chapter 11: Nurturing your health and your baby's continues well beyond pregnancy, so this chapter covers the all-important 'fourth trimester'. We will look at foods to support your healing and help you rebuild your strength after the birth.

Chapter 12: It is well known that breastfeeding can give your baby the best start in life, but by paying attention to your diet you can improve your baby's chances of a healthy future even more. This is a time of high nutrient demand for you, and conserving your energy by making the right food and lifestyle choices is imperative. Discover the best foods to eat during this time, how to lose weight at a healthy rate during breastfeeding and the lifestyle factors that can influence milk production.

Chapter 13: Regular yoga practice can help to support your journey through pregnancy and early motherhood. This short chapter provides you with a gentle 10-minute yoga practice that you can build easily into your daily routine in the comfort of your own home.

Chapter 14: Now learn how to put all your knowledge into practice! This chapter provides a simple navigation chart to help you plan ahead, template menu plans and ideas on meal combinations that focus on the key nutrients detailed in the book. I have also provided delicious recipes by chef Sophie Wright, and practical cooking tips and ideas on how to 'bulk' cook, for easy suppers in the early weeks of parenting and quick after-work meal ideas for the later months.

My hope is that the information provided in this book will offer you accessible, practical and, above all, encouraging advice on the what, when and how to eat during your pregnancy and the early stages of motherhood. Let *Your Pregnancy Nutrition Guide* be a part of the wonderful opportunity that pregnancy is to prioritise your complete well-being, to re-evaluate how you look after yourself in body and mind, and to start building a nurturing relationship with your baby.

Enjoy this precious journey…

CHAPTER 1

NUTRITION TO SUPPORT YOUR FERTILITY

Whether you are planning your first pregnancy or thinking about having another child, trying to conceive naturally or undergoing fertility treatment, the period of time before you conceive gives you a window of opportunity to evaluate your nutrition and general lifestyle.

Small changes to your diet can help you to optimise your 'fertile' ground. This chapter will look at the food and lifestyle choices you and your partner can make to support a healthy conception.

FERTILITY IS PARTNERSHIP

Very often fertility preparation is seen as the preserve of women. In fact, for over half the couples in the UK who experience subfertility (i.e. they are less than normally fertile), it is the result of problems on the male side.

If you and your partner know you want to conceive, you should both try to make some dietary changes three months ahead of that time. During these months, immature eggs, known as oocytes, mature enough to be released during ovulation and sperm cells develop before being ready for ejaculation. Eating a nutritious diet during this time greatly influences the quality and efficiency of this process, and gives you an even greater opportunity to create a healthy pregnancy.

Making dietary changes and improving nutrient stores may also help to correct factors that may be affecting your ability to conceive, such as a low sperm count in men or hormonal imbalances during the menstrual cycle in women.

NUTRITION IS THE FOUNDATION FOR YOU AND YOUR BABY

Studies have shown that couples who have made changes to their diet and lifestyle improved their chances of having a healthy pregnancy and baby by 80 per cent, but research shows that the benefits extend way beyond this. Indeed, how healthy your diet and lifestyle are during the preconception period is now understood to sow the seeds of health for your growing baby in infancy, such as reducing the risk of atopic conditions such as asthma and eczema, as well as chronic health conditions in adulthood, such as diabetes.

Eating a healthy diet before you conceive can also influence milk production during breastfeeding and reduce the potential of postnatal depression.

EATING TO SUPPORT YOUR FERTILITY JOURNEY

- **Eat protein with every meal.** Protein provides the building blocks of the body and is especially important for hormone production and healthy cell development. Good sources of protein include free-range poultry, eggs, yoghurt, fish such as wild salmon and trout, lentils, nuts, seeds, quinoa and grass-fed red meats. If you are vegetarian or vegan, combining pulses and grains provides the optimum amount of vegetarian protein (see page 98). High-protein sources are ideal providers of iron and of the amino acids L-methionine, L-arginine and Co-enzyme Q10. Pulses are also excellent sources of folate (see page 49).
- **Eat healthy fats with every meal.** Healthy fats are vitally important for health and fertility as they support hormone production and healthy cell formation. You will find them in avocado, linseed oil, nuts, seeds and fresh oily fish. However,

limit oily fish to three portions a week because they may contain pollutants that could affect fertility if consumed in high amounts. These food sources are also excellent sources of vitamin E, vitamin D and important minerals, such as chromium and selenium.

- **Eat wholefoods.** Eat as close to nature as was intended by choosing whole grains such as brown rice, red rice, wild rice, quinoa, millet, buckwheat, rye and oats. These are also excellent sources of the B vitamin family, including B12, and minerals such as manganese, zinc and chromium.

- **Eat a rainbow every day.** Eating a colourful variety of fruit and vegetables each day naturally increases your intake of important antioxidants and phytochemicals shown to support preconceptual health, such as beta-carotene from carrots, sweet potatoes and squashes. Adding spices, such as turmeric and ginger, to your cooking is also an excellent way to achieve this 'rainbow'.

- **Eat green leafy vegetables.** As well as being an excellent source of folate, green leafy vegetables provide a great source of fibre for healthy digestion, which helps to prevent hormonal imbalances. Steam them to retain their nutrients. Increase your intake by using them to make juices, soups and smoothies.

- **Eat every four hours.** Eating at regular intervals supports blood-sugar control. Make eating breakfast a priority because this sets up your body well for the day.

- **Eat mindfully.** Digestion begins in the mouth and eating too quickly can reduce your ability to absorb and use the nutrients the food provides. Equally, eating slowly allows the body the time it needs to register its own appetite signals, making it less likely that you will overeat.

- **Eat seasonally if possible.** Seasonal food grown in sync with nature's cycle can improve the nutrient value of the food. Eating seasonally also means eating warmer foods in the colder, damper winter and autumn days, and lighter, less-cooked foods in the warmer, brighter summer and spring days.

FOODS TO BE MINDFUL OF

- **Sushi.** This is a common source of trace metals, such as mercury, so eat in moderation, in line with the oily fish advice on page 9.
- **Sugar.** Sugar robs vital nutrients from bodily stores and can activate a 'fight or flight' stress response. Sugar is not only found in the obvious foods, such as cakes, biscuits and pastries, so read the labels on foods such as healthy-looking cereals and yoghurts. Look for hidden sugars with names such as maltose, dextrose, high fructose and corn syrup. Substitute sugar with healthier alternatives, such as small amounts of raw or manuka honey, or agave syrup.
- **Trans fats.** These fats have been shown to have a detrimental effect on many aspects of health. Foods rich in this type of fat include chips, fried foods, many ready meals, pre-packaged popcorn, biscuits, mayonnaise, margarines and many pre-prepared salad dressings. Eating a diet high in trans fats can reduce how well your body uses the group of essential fats called omega-3 (see page 13). In essence, it is advisable to remove or significantly reduce your intake of these damaged and damaging fats.

DO YOU NEED SUPPLEMENTS?

It is now medically accepted that certain vitamins and minerals can increase your chances of getting and staying pregnant by supporting hormone balance, as well as healthy egg and sperm development. However, increasingly research is showing us that today's environment is not as fertile-friendly for both plant and human as it once was. Many of the foods we eat have been grown on exhausted soil, intensively farmed, picked before they are ripe and transported many miles from source before reaching our plates. As a result, a large proportion of our food is lacking in much-needed trace minerals and vitamins.

Studies have shown that couples who took nutritional supplements to support a healthy diet, had quicker conception rates than those who did not. Below are the nutrients that have been shown to support fertility in both men and women, so look for them when choosing your fertility supplement.

- **B vitamins**. The entire B vitamin family is important during conception and pregnancy. However, vitamin B6 has been shown to support cycle regularity and redress imbalances in hormonal conditions such as fibroids, endometriosis and PMS. Research has shown that giving B6 to women who have trouble conceiving increases fertility. Vitamin B12 has been shown to improve low sperm count and reduce blood stickiness (this is where the blood is thicker than normal and can hinder blood flow).
- **Zinc.** Contributes to normal fertility and reproduction, cell division and protection of cells from general wear and tear. Zinc also contributes to normal DNA synthesis – the genetic material that forms the basis of all of us. Zinc deficiency is common (especially in those women with a history of taking the contraceptive pill) and can affect sperm and egg production.
- **L-methionine.** All amino acids perform a vital role in good health and egg production. However, L-methionine is an essential amino acid that plays a role in hormone stability and therefore supports a regular menstrual cycle. It also protects cellular DNA from damage in the months before you conceive.
- **Beta-carotene.** Because of its status as a fat-soluble nutrient, there has been concern about excess intake of vitamin A in the form of retinol during pregnancy. The vegetable source of vitamin A, beta-carotene, is converted to vitamin A in the body as and when your body needs it, so there is no risk of an excess amount being produced. The corpus luteum, a hormonal structure that produces progesterone after a woman has ovulated, has the highest concentration of beta-carotene in the body and

beta-carotene can influence cycle regularity and the early stages of pregnancy.

- **Vitamin D.** The latest research has demonstrated how important sufficient vitamin D is for a healthy conception and pregnancy, as well as to reduce the risk of gestational diabetes (see page 117). Getting enough vitamin D can be hard through diet and sunshine alone (especially if you live in the northern hemisphere) and so supplements can be a good support.

- **Vitamin E.** This is another antioxidant shown to benefit fertility in both men and women. Supplementing with vitamin E during IVF treatment has been found to improve fertilisation rates.

- **Selenium.** A healthy level of this trace mineral has been shown to improve low sperm count and healthy sperm formation. As an antioxidant it also reduces the risk of miscarriage caused by chromosomal abnormalities.

- **Folic acid.** Along with other members of the B vitamin family, such as vitamin B12, folic acid is used to produce the important genetic material of the egg and the sperm in the three months prior to conception. Folic acid is one part of this group of folates and deficiency in this has been linked to a developmental abnormality known as a neural tube defect (such as spina bifida), which arises between the 24th to 28th day after conception. Supplementation in the three months before you conceive and during the first 12 weeks of pregnancy reduces this risk by 70 per cent, as well as reducing the risk of 'small for gestational age' babies, and cleft lip and palate. The recommendation is for folate to be taken in the 12 weeks prior to conception because once you are pregnant your baby's supply of folate is drawn from the reserves you have built up over the three months before you conceive.

- **Vitamin C.** This is an antioxidant shown to reduce excess histamine, which has been shown to reduce the body's production of cervical mucus. This mucus supports the sperm in reaching the cervix. Vitamin C also acts as a protectant against sperm damage.

- **Chromium & inositol.** These lesser-known nutrients play a role in blood sugar management. Imbalances in blood sugar create a 'stress' response in the body (see page 25).
- **Choline.** This member of the B vitamin family supports normal liver function and how well your body breaks down fats. Liver health significantly affects hormone balance in both men and women. Choline also plays a central role in the unborn baby's brain development.
- **Co-enzyme Q10.** Recent research has shown that Co-enzyme Q10 protects eggs and sperm from damage, as well as supporting healthy cell division in the first stages of pregnancy.
- **Omega-3 fatty acids.** These essential fats support hormone balance and the absorption of fat-soluble nutrients, such as vitamins E, D and K. They also form a large part of the heads of sperm and can therefore influence sperm quality and mobility.

Chapter 12 will give you more information on how to choose quality supplements.

BEYOND NUTRITION: THE INFLUENCE OF LIFESTYLE CHOICES

Becoming as healthy as possible before you conceive is about nourishing your mind as well as your body.

STRESS

Stress is not the preserve of the overworked, as often thought. Factors such as under-achieving, dissatisfaction with where you are in your life, and exercising too little or too much, are all potential 'stressors' to the body. Whatever the reason for your stress, following the nutritional advice in this book can improve how well your body responds to it.

When you are stressed, your body adopts a 'fight or flight' response. This triggers the release of the stress hormones cortisol and adrenaline, which affects digestion, blood pressure, circulation and brain function, and, over time, other areas of health such as hormone balance and nutrient levels.

Teaching yourself to relax, whether by doing yoga (see Chapter 13), massage, meditation or making small tweaks to your everyday routine, such as walking in your lunch hour or going to bed earlier, can provide opportunities to unwind. This is especially helpful during the fertility journey but also during pregnancy and parenthood.

CAFFEINE

Caffeine, especially in the form of coffee, has been shown to have a direct effect on fertility in some men and women. Although government guidelines suggest an intake of 200 mg of caffeine a day (the equivalent of two cups of instant coffee) is regarded as unharmful, studies have shown that drinking as little as one cup of coffee a day can decrease fertility and increase the risk of miscarriage by up to 50 per cent. Caffeine has been found to adversely affect sperm count and motility, and increase sperm abnormalities.

As well as coffee, caffeine is found in tea and fizzy drinks. There is also research into other ingredients found in these drinks, such as the stimulant theobromine, which is also present in decaffeinated versions. If you are trying to conceive, I recommend that you and your partner reduce your consumption of caffeine-containing and decaffeinated drinks, including coffee, colas, diet colas, chocolate, and tea.

ALCOHOL

Alcohol can affect both male and female fertility. The *British Medical Journal* reported that women who had fewer than five units of alcohol a week were twice as likely to become pregnant in a six-month period than those women who drank more than this.

Current recommendations by the Food Standards Agency (FSA) suggest limiting alcohol intake altogether during the preconception period and, if you do drink, have no more than 1–2 units (see page 82) once a week.

In men, alcohol can affect sperm count, motility and quality, and I recommend drinking fewer than four units per week.

Additionally, alcohol can affect hormone balance, as well as reducing nutrient stores of key minerals for fertility, such as zinc (see page 11).

There are times when a having a lovely glass of wine can be part of a balanced lifestyle – when you are celebrating a special occasion, for example – but my advice is to treat alcohol mindfully. Respect the research highlighted above and, when you do drink alcohol, never do so on an empty stomach – this can adversely affect how well your body responds to and metabolises it.

ENVIRONMENTAL FACTORS

Environmental exposure to toxins from pesticides and plastics has been shown to impact on hormone balance and sperm production. The main culprit is a group of chemicals called xenoestrogens, which have a similar structure to the natural hormone oestrogen and contribute to hormonal imbalance. One of the best ways to eliminate an excess intake of these in the months before you conceive is to eat organic produce – particularly grains, fruit and vegetables you do not peel, such as berries and broccoli – as well as meat and dairy.

Toxic metals such as mercury and lead may also impact fertility in both men and women. These can be found in pesticides, heavy consumption of oily fish (see page 9), and there is a small amount in amalgam dental fillings. Additionally, exposure to other chemicals and toxic metals found in cigarettes, have also been shown to impact on healthy development of the unborn baby. This is the ideal time to find the support you need to give up smoking for both you, your baby and your partner.

Medication can influence our nutrient levels too. For example, metformin, a drug given to people with Type 2 diabetes, can reduce stores of vitamin B12, the contraceptive pill can reduce vitamin B6 and healthy bacteria in the gut, and statin medication for high cholesterol reduces Co-enzyme Q10 stores.

For more information on these important environmental factors, I recommend you look at the website for foresight preconception (see page 214).

GOOD LIVER HEALTH:
THE ENGINE ROOM

The hormonal balance needed for fertility depends on good liver function. Aside from its daily task of detoxifying substances, such as caffeine and environmental toxins, the liver also chemically alters an excess of or used hormones. If this process does not happen effectively, hormonal imbalances can occur affecting fertility and other health concerns such as endometriosis, acne, premenstrual syndrome (PMS) and polycystic ovary syndrome (PCOS). A gentle liver-cleansing programme with the help of a nutritional therapist or naturopath prior to conception can be a great starting point for some women and men.

• • •

It's my heartfelt belief that building a relationship with your baby can start before you conceive. Investing in and caring for your health during the preconception period will provide your baby with a nutrient-rich environment in which to thrive from day one of pregnancy. It is the window of opportunity for you to start building the nutrient reserves for your experience of a healthy pregnancy too, to minimise your experience of common pregnancy ailments and make pregnancy the enjoyable, blossoming journey that it can be.

CHAPTER 2

YOU AND YOUR BABY ARE WHAT YOU EAT

Your unborn baby begins to develop at conception. At the moment the sperm penetrates the egg, a new organism is created with its own unique combination of over 20,000 genes. Development from this moment and during the first trimester is rapid and quite miraculous – by day 23 your baby's heart has formed. I firmly believe that you become a mother not when your baby is placed into your arms for the first time, but at the moment of conception. Nurturing your baby begins from this day on and is a life-changing and sometimes daunting responsibility. The first nurturing responsibility is to grow your baby from seed to bump to a healthy newborn.

GETTING IT RIGHT

All pregnant women share a common desire: to have a healthy baby. During this formative time they just want to get things right and to know that they have done everything within their power to achieve it. Many of us know that eating well during pregnancy is a good thing – both for your baby's health, as well as your own. Looking after your own well-being can only have a positive effect on your unborn child. Eating well is also a wonderful opportunity to begin the nurturing relationship that will continue once your child is born. It is a very powerful and demanding time for your body and feeding it with the right fuel is incredibly important.

Nutrition before conception and during pregnancy has been of great interest to researchers for some time. More recently, however, research has looked more deeply into the impact of diet during pregnancy and its effects on long-term health. It is such an important area that it became a subject of research for the British Nutrition Foundation Task Force in 2013.

Research has shown that the quality of a mother's diet before she conceives and during pregnancy produces lifelong effects that can improve her baby's resistance to infection and degenerative disease later in life. Eating well in pregnancy is thought not only to benefit that baby but her subsequent children too. It is a comforting thought that by eating a healthy and nutritious diet you are supporting your baby's future health and that of her children too.

Not only has research confirmed the importance of good nutrition in pregnancy, but the link between nutrition and health has generated some incredible and ground-breaking findings. The most significant of these are foetal programming and epigenetics, which I explain below. Both areas of research have totally transformed the way we look at inherited 'good' or 'bad' health.

FOETAL PROGRAMMING

Foetal programming is defined as a process whereby an environmental stimulus, such as nutrient deficiencies (for example, folate deficiency – see page 49), at a critical phase of development, result in long-term changes in the development of the baby while in the womb. This concept was introduced by Professor David Barker and his colleagues at the University of Southampton in 1989. His ground-breaking work took research into the development of human disease to another level, proposing that a woman's diet and body composition at the time of conception and during pregnancy have important effects on the subsequent health of her children.

EPIGENETICS

A growing body of evidence is emerging on the role of 'epigenetics' while the baby is growing in the womb. In simple terms, this is the study of how environmental factors such as diet, stress and pollutants can affect how your genes affect your health. It is thought that these factors can even turn certain genes on and off. This challenges previous thinking that genetics were something we couldn't change – for example, that you are either genetically susceptible to breast cancer or you are not. Research is now discovering that although these genes can be turned on with poor eating habits, we can also turn off potentially destructive genes by eating a healthy diet. It is believed that this 'epigenetic memory' is passed to the next generation through sperm and eggs, and during development when in the womb. This is empowering information for those trying to conceive and for pregnant women. If a mother eats a nutritious diet during this sensitive period, she can produce positive changes to her baby's physiology and genetic expression – how her genes affect her health. For example, some individuals show greater resistance to the effects of stressors in adult life as a result of positive experiences in early life, which can include good nutrition.

An expectant mother's diet has been shown to have as much as a 62 per cent effect on her unborn baby's development, with only 20 per cent being influenced by maternal genes and 18 per cent from the baby's genes itself. What these findings mean is that mothers can have a greater influence on the health of their unborn child than was previously understood. This evidence is of vital importance because from conception to six months of age, babies are entirely dependent on their mother for all nutrition, initially via the placenta and then ideally through exclusive breastfeeding for six months. This period of 15 months (about 500 days) – from conception through to the end of breastfeeding – is the most important and vulnerable in a child's life and the perfect opportunity for you to have some control over the future health of your child. Nutrients and macronutrients (fats, carbohydrates and proteins) from your diet are a pivotal part this crucial development of your growing baby. This initial stage of rapid development is reliant on your nutritional status, drawing on the folate or vitamin B12, for example, that you have built up in the months before you conceived.

NATURE AT WORK

Good nutrition is so important that, at a time of extreme shortage, the reproductive system can shut down, halting menstruation and a woman's ability to reproduce. Pregnancy is yet another example of nature's brilliance. This shutdown is instinctive: a bodily reaction that occurs to avoid the risk of an undernourished or sick baby in the womb. Of course, we are talking about extreme nutrient deficiency here, but this mechanism further illustrates the connection between the mother's nutrient stores and the baby's development.

Not everyone is convinced of the vital importance of nutrition during pregnancy. Sceptics often argue that there are many cultures where women live in poor conditions with little access to wholesome food, yet still give birth to seemingly healthy babies. However, studies have shown that babies born from these malnourished women are often sick. An example of this is the study of the Dutch 'Hunger Winter' that occurred between 1944–1945, during the Second World War, which highlighted the 'critical window' of nutrition in early pregnancy. It was clear from this study that exposure to a nutrient-rich diet, especially during the first trimester, significantly improves a baby's health after birth, enabling her to balance blood-sugar levels (see page 24), reducing the risk of high blood pressure, giving her greater tolerance of stress in later life and healthy mental development. Those women who were in the last trimester of pregnancy limited their increased risk to glucose intolerance, hypertension and impaired insulin secretion. Interestingly, exposure to famine in early pregnancy was also associated with differences in food choices later in life. The babies born during the famine were twice as likely to choose high-fat foods than those that were not exposed to dietary restrictions in the womb.

The women in the research detailed above are an extreme example of poverty and they lived during a time of incredible emotional and physical stress. With the food choices we have today, this research can be seen as empowering, giving you the information you need to nourish your baby in the womb as best you can, while increasing the chances of your child's good health in their future. You can do a lot with small, sustainable changes that will greatly nourish you and improve your baby's nutritional foundation.

SUPPORTING A HEALTHY BIRTH WEIGHT

One of the key roles good nutrition plays in the growth of your unborn baby is the development of a healthy birth weight. Low birth weight is classified as any baby weighing under 2.5 kg (5½ lb). Low birth weight is associated with a greater risk of many health conditions, including asthma and autism. Mother Nature is very clever and, in fact, during mid-pregnancy, if there is mild nutritional deficiency, the placenta actually grows to maintain the nutrient supply from the mother. If this deficiency continues, the unborn baby's growth can be affected. Later on in pregnancy, in the third trimester, if nutritional deficiency occurs then growth will be slow but then rapidly restored when good nutrition is resumed. However, if nutritional deficiency is constant over the pregnancy then slow growth is predicted to continue even after the baby has been born.

Genetic factors, such as parental height and weight, may also play a role in determining newborn birth weight. Babies who are a low birth weight because of their genes are not at a higher risk of the health conditions detailed above.

Over the last decade, the overall proportion of babies in England and Wales who are of low birth weight has remained relatively unchanged at approximately 7 per cent. We fall just behind Thailand, Romania and Swaziland, leaving us statistically the third worst in Europe. This is quite shocking considering our relative affluence and access to food. In mothers who gave birth to low birth weight babies, 43 out of 44 nutrients measured in the mothers were significantly below those of mothers whose babies fell within the normal range. So why, when we have an increasing awareness of the importance of nutrition, do we continue to have such a bad record on low birth weight here in the UK? Evidence suggests it may have a lot to do with our Western diet and lifestyle. Our food is produced on a large scale and is becoming what chef Doug McMaster calls 'de-natured', bleached and highly processed. Modern production and an increased use of medication all deplete the nutrients found in our food.

OUR WESTERN DIETS

The rapid change in food manufacturing practices over the last 50 years has created a society that is progressively in danger of losing touch with 'real food'. Our busy lifestyles can have an immense effect on our eating habits and nutrient intake, meaning that the reality of sitting down to a delicious plate of steamed seasonal vegetables, lean proteins and whole grains seems far from simple. Equally, statistics show that we can no longer rely on our food to supply us with the full range and quantity of the vital nutrients we require for optimum health. As long ago as 1936, the US Senate recognised the growing depletion of nutrients in our soils worldwide and published a report stating that:

The alarming fact is that foods (fruit, vegetables and grains) are now being raised on millions of acres of land that no longer contain enough of certain minerals and are therefore starving us – no matter how much of them we eat. No man of today can eat enough fruit and vegetables to supply his system with the minerals he requires for perfect health.

US soil is now estimated to be between 55–85 per cent less nutrient-rich than it was 60 years ago, meaning that the vital vitamins and minerals in our 'fresh' fruit and vegetables have been greatly depleted. Even 'healthier' organic food can be up to 10 times less nutritious than before. This problem is not unique to the US and over a decade ago a report from the Department for Environment, Food & Rural Affairs (DEFRA) stated that the trace minerals in UK fruit and vegetables had fallen by over 76 per cent. Further to this, a study by the *British Food Journal* reported that in the last 50 years the potato has suffered substantial nutrient losses, including 100 per cent of vitamin A content, 57 per cent of vitamin C, 28 per cent of calcium and 50 per cent of riboflavin.

Decades of intensive farming and a global market of importation and exportation has meant that fruit and vegetables are being picked before they are ripe, significantly reducing their nutritional value. This is supported by the work of independent researcher Ann-Marie Mayer, who examined nutrient data in two 'time points', separated by approximately 50 years. She published in the UK government's *Composition of Foods* that the reduction in mineral content of the soil is statistically significant.

• • •

The state of the global food industry may be bleak, but with an increased knowledge of nutrition and how to get the most from your food, you can still provide your unborn baby with all the vitamins needed for a healthy future. By eating locally sourced, seasonal food and by taking the recommended supplements, you can improve your own well-being and that of your child. In Chapter 7, I will be examining supplements and their role in pregnancy in much more detail.

CHAPTER 3

BUILDING YOUR NUTRITION IN PREGNANCY

Once you become pregnant, it is not a case of eating for two but caring for two. Before becoming pregnant, you may have skipped breakfast or eaten unhealthy snacks to fill a gap between meals. Such habits will have been affecting your health without you even realising it. Becoming pregnant is an opportunity for you to develop an awareness of the effects that your usual eating habits can have on your health, most especially the importance of balancing your blood sugar for yourself and your growing baby. I hope that this chapter will help you to embrace good eating patterns and practices as soon as you fall pregnant, if not before.

BALANCING YOUR BLOOD SUGAR

Stabilising your blood sugar is a key part of healthy eating during pregnancy. It will support your energy levels, reduce the incidence of symptoms such as morning sickness (see page 104), reduce the risk of gestational diabetes (see page 117) and support your body's response to the hormonal changes that occur. In the first trimester, too much blood sugar instability can slow growth, whereas in the last trimester, in the form of gestational diabetes, it can accelerate growth giving the baby a high birth weight. This is just as much of a concern as a low birth weight (see page 21).

Keeping your blood sugar balanced is a matter of survival so your body has a well-tuned system of maintaining it, sometimes at the cost of other bodily functions. There is a common analogy used by nutritional therapists, including myself, which compares the blood-sugar mechanism to that of a thermostat that controls a central heating system. A thermostat is acutely sensitive to when the temperature rises or falls, and in the same way your body's finely tuned 'thermostat' clicks on when your blood sugar is too high or low.

When you eat, your food is broken down into glucose and absorbed into the bloodstream via the gut. This creates a 'surge' of glucose in the bloodstream that is then fed into the cells, especially your energy-hungry brain cells, to produce energy and, in the case of pregnancy, to fuel the growth of your baby. However, if you eat foods that produce a 'surge' of glucose that is more than your body needs, it triggers a greater release of the hormone insulin from the pancreas. Insulin transports the glucose, taking it to be transformed into glycogen, and then stores it away in the liver or muscles for another time. The degree to which this occurs is influenced by what you eat and drink. If you are not eating properly, your blood-sugar levels zoom up and down chaotically. This causes symptoms such as mood swings, intense cravings and bingeing, usually on the wrong sort of sugary foods.

When blood sugar drops too low, it triggers the release of adrenaline and glucagon, which initiate an immediate release of the glycogen stored in the liver or muscles. This takes precious stored energy away from the development of your baby and is the reason why blood sugar disruption is associated with lower birth weight babies. If blood sugar remains low for a period of time, a condition called hypoglycaemia can occur and you can experience dizziness, heart palpitations, agitation, fatigue, excessive sweating, thirst and an intense need to eat something. The release of adrenaline in response to this drop can interfere with the uptake of progesterone, the sex hormone that 'holds' the pregnancy in the early weeks. For this reason, stabilising blood-sugar levels has been shown to reduce the risk of miscarriage.

SIMPLE WAYS TO BALANCE YOUR BLOOD SUGAR

The body is an incredibly complex machine, but treating it right doesn't have to be overwhelming. By following a few simple rules and establishing some good habits, it can become much easier to balance your blood sugar, not only during pregnancy but throughout the rest of your life. The following guidelines will help you to lay the right foundations on which to build a nutrient-dense pregnancy diet that balances your blood-sugar levels throughout the next nine months:

- Eat every three hours. During the first trimester, and indeed during the entire pregnancy, eating smaller meals regularly during the day will support your appetite.
- Swap simple carbohydrates for 'complex' carbohydrates (see page 36).
- Eat a source of protein, complex carbohydrates and healthy fats at each meal and snack (see Chapter 14 for meal plans and recipes).
- Always eat breakfast.
- Minimise or preferably avoid eating processed foods and foods containing added sugar.
- Avoid sugary fizzy drinks or 'diet' varieties.
- Aim for a rainbow of colourful vegetables on your plate at every meal to increase the variety of nutrients. Vegetables also contain high amounts of water and fibre. Spices and herbs add colour, too, so add these to your food to make them look more appealing and appetising, and to improve the nutrient value of your meal.
- Keep hydrated: about 6–8 glasses of water are needed for most adults and while you are pregnant or breastfeeding you will likely find that you need more.
- Eat slowly. Savour your food and give it the full attention it requires. Chewing your food is the second significant part of digestion (thinking of and smelling food is the first step!). As much as 30–40 per cent of our digestive response to food comes from having 'awareness' when we eat. This simply means that if

we do not concentrate on our food or eat mindfully, our ability to digest the food can be reduced by up to 40 per cent.

MAXIMISE NUTRITION

The way that you shop for, or cook, your food can help you to maximise nutritious eating. For example, shopping for fresh fruit and vegetables two or three times a week is better than making one big purchase. Fruit and vegetables lose their nutrient value fairly quickly as they age, so keeping them as fresh as possible can make a difference. When fruit becomes too 'soft' the fruit sugars increase, so try to eat fruit at its peak of ripeness. When it isn't possible to buy fresh fruit and vegetables, opt for frozen rather than tinned. Some frozen foods, such as peas and berries, contain comparable nutrient levels to the fresh variety but others, such as broccoli and beans, do not.

Keeping the skin on your vegetables or fruit can also affect its nutrient value for you and your baby. For most fruit and vegetables, the nutrients are stored just under the 'zest' and the skins are also a great source of fibre. So instead of peeling, scrub them and cook them with their skins on.

When cooking your vegetables, choose steaming rather than boiling. The steaming process helps the food to retain its nutrients, whereas boiling causes the nutrients to leach into the water. If you do boil, use as little water as possible and save this water to use in soups and sauces. Don't throw away the stems either! The stems of vegetables, such as broccoli, are packed with nutrients but are often thrown away. Instead, use these to make soups and juices.

PREPARING FRUIT AND VEGETABLES

Once fruit and vegetables are cut, they start to lose their nutrient content. Chop them only when you are ready to cook them, if possible.

SEASONAL EATING

During my pregnancies, I became acutely aware of the natural 'cycle of life' that is all around us, in nature but also in our food. Pregnancy is a true expression of this cycle and so it seems apt that during this time you should eat seasonally where you can. Foods that are grown in season tend to be picked when they are ripe, which increases the nutrient value. It also means that we are supplied with the right balance of nutrients at the time that we need them; Mother Nature cleverly provides vegetables rich in carotenes for immune support in the autumn, for example. In the colder months, choose warming soups and roasted root vegetables and in the warmer months choose lighter salads and meals. Soups, juices and smoothies are an excellent way of packing in the nutrients, although juices and smoothies also have their drawbacks (see page 54). I firmly believe that we should eat foods that are warm in the colder months and foods that are cooler in the warmer months. According to naturopathic and Traditional Chinese Medicine principles, eating in this way also supports digestion

During the autumn and winter seasons, revive the slow cooker. Low temperatures preserve many of the essential nutrients found in meat. It can also make the meat more digestible without destroying the benefits of the amino acids (see page 33) needed for your baby's growth. Aside from this, the slow cooker is a practical, cost-efficient way of having a meal ready at the end of the day.

CALORIE COUNTING

We have all heard of new mums complaining that they are unable to 'shift' the baby weight or are still in maternity jeans well beyond giving birth. As a result, many mums-to-be are fearful of gaining too much weight during pregnancy. If, however, you eat a well-balanced, wholesome diet throughout your pregnancy, your weight gain should be proportionate to your needs and those of your baby and therefore you can avoid any need to 'diet' after your baby is born.

During the first trimester, while your body is getting used to these growing demands of fuel, you may find that your appetite changes. Although officially you need no extra calories in this trimester, let your appetite be your guide as you may not have been eating enough daily fuel prior to pregnancy. An increase in your appetite is also a mechanism to indicate areas of your nutrition that your body needs to top up. If you are eating a well-balanced diet of macronutrients and micronutrients (see Chapters 4 and 5), then these cravings are likely to be less. This balanced eating is also vital for reducing the unwanted symptoms of early pregnancy, such as morning sickness and tiredness (see Chapter 9).

The total number of calories used to fuel your nine months of pregnancy is estimated to be 76,000, and you might assume that you need a significantly higher calorie intake. In fact, providing you were eating sufficient calories before you were pregnant, you do not need any additional calories in the first trimester. You then need 200 extra calories a day in the second trimester and 400 extra a day in the third trimester. Your body's use of calories is extremely efficient during pregnancy and, therefore, as long as you are eating nutrient-dense food, such as lean proteins and green leafy vegetables, and not 'empty foods' such as sugary, white flour products, and are not diabetic, you do not need to be overly concerned with calorie counting. Pregnancy is not the time to simply focus on calories. Instead focus on eating nutrient-dense, whole foods that can balance the body and enrich you. Even after giving birth calories should not be the main focus of your diet (see Chapter 11). I do not recommend dieting at all in the early stages of new motherhood; instead the focus should still be on eating well to recover and heal from the birth and support the energy-demanding fourth trimester.

CREATING A HEALTHY 'MIND-SET'

Eating in a way that nourishes you and your baby does not need to be obsessive. In fact, quite the opposite. Healthy eating is an emotional and physical experience, involving all the senses. Taking the time to enjoy your food and relax around mealtimes can affect how well your food is used by your body. For many the sense of 'balance' when choosing food has been lost. Instead their food choices are governed by calories or adverts suggesting that they will feel or look better if they eat a branded food. Listening to your body has taken a back seat and instead many women are hounded by feelings of guilt or shame about the foods they eat: 'Will this make me fat?'; 'I feel hungry but I shouldn't snack.' The reality is our appetite changes from day to day, often for good reason, and this could not be more true during pregnancy. It is so important for you to listen to your body's needs and provide it and your baby with the most nutrient-dense, nourishing fuel for growth.

• • •

Our children begin learning from us in the very early days, even in the womb, so rediscover your passion for real food now and pass it on to your baby. Think quality over quantity, and find pleasure in experimenting with foods you may not have chosen before. Pregnancy is a great opportunity to begin a better way of eating for life.

CHAPTER 4

MACRONUTRIENTS: THE BUILDING BLOCKS OF YOUR DIET

During the first 12 weeks of pregnancy your baby's growth is rapid, with cell division occurring at a rate of 250,000 per minute! The brain, heart and lungs, among other organs, are developed even before you are six weeks pregnant. It is also at this stage that most of the foundational changes discussed in Chapter 2 occur, when the effect of environmental factors, such as diet, are at their most influential. You and your baby are working incredibly hard and it is not dissimilar to preparing for a marathon!

The guidelines in this chapter will help you to take the foundations of healthy nutrition outlined in Chapter 3 and apply them to your pregnancy diet. This will enable you to avoid unhealthy weight gain, reduce the risk of developing gestational diabetes (see page 117) and encourage the healthy development of your unborn baby, as well as supporting your own health and that of your baby after the birth. The food that you eat affects every cell in your body, which is why healthy eating during pregnancy is so important and can support giving birth to a healthy baby. In these early stages, your nutrition is key.

YOUR BABY'S LIFELINE

During the first 12 weeks of pregnancy, your baby is reliant on the nutritional status of the yolk sac. At 12 weeks, the placenta takes over and nutrients are extracted from your blood to supply the health of your baby. Your baby's growth beyond the first trimester is dependent on a healthy placenta, and the quality of your placenta will be built on the nutrient stores acquired before you conceived and during the first three months of pregnancy. This healthy placenta will optimise the exchange of nutrients and oxygen to your baby for the rest of your pregnancy.

I FEEL SO SICK THAT I CAN HARDLY EAT ANYTHING HEALTHY

Morning sickness affects about 75 per cent of women in early pregnancy and this common pregnancy symptom can limit the amount of healthy foods you want to eat. The good news is that your baby is unlikely to be affected. If you have built up a good storage of nutrients before you became pregnant, your baby will simply draw on these for the first 12 weeks. There are lots of things that you can do to help relieve your symptoms (see page 104).

SMALL STEPS

Many of my clients have reported feeling 'the best they have ever felt' during pregnancy simply by choosing to make small dietary changes. Rather than experiencing swollen ankles and having no energy at nine months, it is possible to feel clear-headed and energetic. And the changes really are small. It is incredible the difference that can be made by, for example, swapping white rice for brown rice, or tinned sweetcorn for fresh broccoli. You do not need to give up all the things you like – having the occasional chocolate bar or sausage will not derail a healthy lifestyle, but being well-informed about food will allow you to make an educated choice. You are likely to find that you enjoy these changes and eating in this way not only because nutritious food can still taste really good, but because it will make you feel so well too.

UNDERSTANDING YOUR FOOD

Nutrient sources can be broken down into two categories: macronutrients and micronutrients. *Macro*nutrients are protein, carbohydrates and fats that provide calories – they are essential to maintaining health and development. *Micro*nutrients are vitamins and minerals, such as magnesium or vitamin D. All micronutrients, although needed in smaller amounts, have an important role in the body. Some of these vitamins and minerals can be made by the body, but others need to be obtained through our food and by eating macronutrients.

Not all food is created equal and knowing which food is the most nourishing choice can sometimes be a minefield. This chapter and the following chapter will help you to understand what those better choices are, why we need these macronutrients and micronutrients, where you can find them and when you may need them during the pregnancy.

PROTEIN

All protein is made up of amino acids. These amino acids are the basic building blocks of all human tissue so, as you can imagine, protein is very important when building a new human being! Protein is needed for the growth of your unborn baby and the placenta, as well as to support the hormonal changes that occur during pregnancy. Amino acids also form the enzymes necessary for the digestive processes and these processes can affect how well you absorb other nutrients from your food. Protein continues to be of great importance after the birth as it is also needed for the production of breast milk.

Nine amino acids are categorised as 'essential' as you cannot make them in the human body and therefore need to get them from your diet. It is these 'essential' amino acids that are particularly important during pregnancy. The amino acid tryptophan is one of these essential amino acids. It is needed to generate the production of serotonin, your body's natural 'feel good' chemical, and is critical for your developing baby. It is thought to be produced by the placenta during pregnancy for supporting brain, heart and pancreatic development, and may play a role in reducing the brain alterations associated with autism, although this requires further research.

Another group of amino acids is categorised as 'conditional', which means that they are not essential to health, but, during certain times in our life, they become necessary. Pregnancy is one of these occasions. Glycine is one of the amino acids that is conditionally essential during pregnancy. This means that although we are able to make it ourselves, during pregnancy we must also ensure we are getting enough from our food. Food sources are those that are naturally rich in amino acids, such as the skin from meat and bones used to make stock or broths. These foods are also rich in another amino acid, taurine, which plays a role in the neural development of your baby – in fact taurine is present at three times the adult level when your baby is newborn.

Animal products and fish contain the full range of 'essential' amino acids. This does not mean to say they cannot be obtained through a vegetarian or vegan diet. To get a full range of 'essential' amino acids from vegetable sources, you can combine pulses with nuts or seeds, for example (see Chapter 8 for advice on a vegan or vegetarian diet in pregnancy).

WHERE DO I FIND PROTEIN?

Good sources of quality protein include:

● Lean red meat (such as beef and lamb)

- Game
- Fish
- Eggs
- Semi-skimmed or whole milk
- Plain yoghurt
- Pulses (such as chickpeas, cannellini beans and lentils)
- Tofu
- Nuts and seeds

CHOOSE YOUR RED MEAT MINDFULLY

Although red meat is a good source of minerals, including iron and zinc, as well as B vitamins, research has shown that eating more than 70 g (2½ oz) per day poses a greater risk for bowel cancer and other digestive diseases such as diverticulitis. Considering that two average pork sausages is 100 g (3½ oz) and an average portion of bacon is 45 g (1½ oz), it would be easy to eat more than this.

The benefits of red meat can also be affected by how processed it is and there is a world of difference between the red meat found in sausages and ham, and that of a grass-fed lamb chop. When red meat is processed, cured or smoked, it contains sodium nitrate. This helps to turn packaged meat a bright red colour, so that it looks fresh, as well as preserving it so that it has a longer shelf life. Some studies have also drawn an association between sodium nitrate and colorectal cancer but this link is as yet inconclusive. You shouldn't cut red meat out; just eat smaller portions of quality red meat two or three times a week.

HOW MUCH PROTEIN?

Throughout pregnancy and during the breastfeeding period you need to increase your intake of protein to approximately 55 g (2 oz) a day (from 45 g/1½ oz as a non-pregnant woman). This is the equivalent of 220 g (7¾ oz) of chicken or fish, or two medium eggs.

CARBOHYDRATES

Carbohydrates are the main source of energy in our diets and craving this type of food is common in pregnancy. Carbohydrates provide glucose that powers your pregnancy and the growth of your baby. They also provide many of the essential minerals required during pregnancy, such as the B vitamins, including folate and vitamin B12, and the mineral zinc.

Some women shy away from carbohydrate foods, due to concerns that they are 'fattening'. In fact, carbohydrates are often low in fat and high in the minerals needed to support a healthy metabolism. Cravings for carbohydrates during the early stages of pregnancy are common, but it is important to understand that there are two kinds of carbohydrates and they work very differently. Refined carbohydrates (otherwise known as 'simple' carbohydrates) are foods, such as white flour products, many processed breakfast cereals, cakes and biscuits. Then there are unrefined or 'complex' carbohydrates, such as wholewheat, brown rice, millet or rye. It is important to know the difference, especially during pregnancy when maintaining healthy blood-sugar levels (see page 24) is even more important for your health and that of your baby.

SIMPLE OR REFINED CARBOHYDRATES

While it is perfectly healthy to indulge your cravings for unrefined carbohydrates, it is not the case for the 'refined' versions. The more 'refined' a carbohydrate is, the more it acts like pure sugar. This type of carbohydrate is broken down very easily into glucose molecules and can be very quickly used as a source of energy. This may sound good but the reality is very different indeed. Instead, these easily accessed glucose molecules cause a sudden surge of glucose in the bloodstream followed by an equally rapid nosedive. This extreme high and low results in low energy, cravings for sugary foods, weight gain and can leave you at greater risk of gestational diabetes. These foods contain little in the way of nutrients and are in fact termed 'anti-nutrients' by nutritionists – to metabolise them the body has to use up important nutrients such as chromium and B vitamins.

Examples of simple or refined carbohydrates include:

- White caster sugar
- White rice
- White pasta
- White flour and bread
- Packaged biscuits, chocolate, confectionary and cakes
- Fizzy drinks

COMPLEX OR UNREFINED CARBOHYDRATES

Complex carbohydrates provide glucose, but are significantly slower at being broken down. This provides a more sustainable release of energy, supports a healthy weight and can lower the risk of gestational diabetes. When complex carbohydrates are mixed with proteins this effect is even greater – for example, sardines on wholewheat toast or oatcakes with nut butter.

Additionally, complex carbohydrates are a rich source of B vitamins, including B12, folate and vitamin B6, and the minerals iron, magnesium and selenium, which are needed for a healthy immune system. They also supply fibre, another key macronutrient. Fibre helps us to remove unwanted waste products from the gut and reduce constipation, which, as many pregnant women can tell you, is a welcome relief!

WHERE DO I FIND UNREFINED CARBOHYDRATES?

- Wholewheat pasta
- Wholewheat bread
- Bulgur wheat
- Long-grain brown rice
- Spelt
- Rye

BREAKFAST CEREALS

I often say to my clients that to get nutrient value from breakfast cereals, you might as well eat the box. Although this is said tongue-in-cheek, there is also some truth to it. Many of the mainstream breakfast cereals are processed in such a way that much of the goodness is stripped out of the original ingredients. By law, these cereals have to provide a minimum amount of nutrients, so the manufacturers then fortify the cereal with nutrients that might have been taken out in the first place. The cereal is marketed with claims such as 'with added calcium' or 'added folic acid', inferring it has additional health properties. In fact, the cereals now contain synthetic replicas of the food-sourced nutrient they removed. These synthetic replicas are far from the perfect replacement for the original food-bound nutrients and can be harder for our body to assimilate. Be wary of claims such as 'healthy' and 'added nutrients'. Children's cereals are perhaps the worst. So think outside the box, literally, and explore other breakfast options such as oat or millet porridge, avocado on wholemeal toast, or Greek yoghurt and fruit. You can find more breakfast ideas and recipes in Chapter 14.

- Millet
- Oats
- Buckwheat
- Quinoa
- Wholegrain wild rice
- All fruit and vegetables

HOW MUCH CARBOHYDRATE?

Ideally carbohydrates should make up about 60 per cent of your daily calorie intake and be a mix of whole grains, fruit and vegetables.

FATS

There are many misconceptions about fat when it comes to health; the most prominent of which is that fat is bad for you. The reality is that fats are the powerhouse for every cell in your body and that of your baby, too. This is especially so for brain development because over 60 per cent of the brain is made of fat. As we have discovered, the unborn baby's brain goes through significant growth during the first and third trimester. A good supply of healthy fats is therefore crucial for optimum development, and also important to build stores for breastfeeding and your recovery after the birth. In fact, research has shown that improving your intake of the essential fats (also known as omega-3 and omega-6) can reduce the risk of your baby having a low birth weight and of you getting postnatal depression.

I have had the pleasure of working with Professor Michael Crawford on a number of occasions, who is now perhaps the world's leading expert on fats for brain development. Since the 1960s, he has been brilliantly vocal about the essential nature of fat for foetal development; not a popular viewpoint in the era of Jane Fonda and the 'low fat' eating trend.

He says:

> *The brain is largely made of fat (60 per cent) ... The bulk of brain division and its capacity is built early in pregnancy. Moreover, brain development is dependent on maternal health, DHA intake and nutrition.*

Eating fats is also important to support your intake of fat-soluble vitamins A, D, E and K, as well as the fat-soluble plant compounds such as carotenes that can support the immune system.

There are three types of fat that we can obtain from the diet. These are saturated, monounsaturated and polyunsaturated. However, as with carbohydrates, there are significant health differences between the different categories of fats.

SATURATED FATS

Animal products such as meat and dairy products are the main source of saturated fats and are solid at room temperature. Saturated fats have been rather underappreciated in my view, mostly due to the incorrect but very bad press that all saturated fats are harmful. Although they are a fat to be more mindful of than some of the others, small amounts can actually support health. Arachidonic acid (AA) found in saturated fats is actually essential for skin health, immune response, the strength of the gut lining and brain function as your baby develops. However your body can produce small amounts of saturated fat itself, so these are not essential to find in the diet. Healthy sources of saturated fats include coconut oil and egg yolks, both of which have been shown to have health benefits when eaten moderately.

MONOUNSATURATED FATS

These are not essential to health but have been associated with some health benefits and can be a regular part of your healthy

TRANS FATS

Trans fats (also called hydrogenated fats) are those (mainly vegetable fats) that have gone through a chemical process that turns them from liquids into solid. This process damages the structure of the fat, changing them from their more healthy unsaturated nature to a less desirable trans fat structure, and has been linked to a number of health concerns, including high cholesterol and fertility issues. Trans fats also serve to inhibit your body's use of the essential fats omega-3. Thankfully many food manufacturers are voluntarily taking greater responsibility over this area of food production and either stating the inclusion of trans fats in their ingredients lists or avoiding their use completely. These fats are found in fast food, fried foods, crisps, cakes, biscuits and margarine.

pregnancy diet. Examples are olive oil, rapeseed oil, avocados and nuts, including walnuts, almonds, cashews and pistachios.

POLYUNSATURATED FATS (PUFAS)

PUFAs, also known as 'essential fatty acids', cannot be made by your body and it is therefore essential to obtain them from your diet. They are a vital component of every cell in the body, are needed to balance hormones, insulate nerve cells and keep the skin supple (think stretch marks). This group of fats includes omega-3 (found in vegetable oils, such as rapeseed, and in flaxseed, nuts, seeds and oily fish, such as wild salmon, trout or sardines), and omega-6 (found in vegetable oils, such as sunflower oil). We can easily find omega-6 in our diet; in fact, arguably we eat too many of these, but omega-3 is consumed a lot less.

Omega-3 from fish sources provides two important fatty acids for pregnancy known as eicosapentaenoic acid (EPA) and docosahexaenoic acid (DHA). These fatty acids are vital building blocks for brain and nerve development for your unborn baby, and for eye and brain development in early infancy. There has been a considerable amount of research into the role of DHA and how insufficient levels can lead to premature births and low birth weight. It is estimated that during pregnancy a baby accumulates at least 10 g of DHA, 6–7 g of which is in the last trimester, mainly for brain development.

These fatty acids, EPA and DHA, do not need converting to be active in the body. However, the fatty acids found in nuts, seeds and vegetable oils do need to be converted. Zinc, magnesium, calcium and B vitamins support this conversion, so keeping healthy levels of these is also important (see Chapter 5). Stress, a high-sugar diet, caffeine, and trans or hydrogenated fats (see page 41) can also reduce your body's ability to convert these fatty acids.

BUTTER

Clients of mine are often surprised when I suggest using butter in their diet. I think poor old butter has had a rough deal and been rather overshadowed by the fat scandal. However, many of the alternatives are far from healthy. A little, preferably unsalted, organic or grass-fed, butter does little harm and can, in fact, be a great addition to the diet as it is rich in the fat-soluble nutrients vitamins A, D, E and K, as well as selenium, copper, zinc and chromium. It also provides iodine, critical for healthy thyroid function, and lecithin, needed for brain development. Choose solid, traditional butter rather than 'butter spreads'.

HOW MUCH FAT?

Fats shouldn't make up more than 35 per cent of your calorie intake per day (about 30 g/1 oz). Ideally, the majority should come from omega-3, such as oily fish, and a moderate amount from monounsaturated fats, such as olive oil, and saturated fats found in animal fat and dairy. The expert panel at the European Commission recommends at least 200 mg of DHA a day, but there is a significant body of research to show that around 300–400 mg of DHA per day, the equivalent of around 15 g (½ oz) of wild salmon, is optimum during pregnancy and breastfeeding, and I agree with this. This level of fish intake can also increase cases of pregnancies reaching full term. This intake was seen to be so important that the report recommended that dietary inadequacy of DHA should be screened for during pregnancy. However, there are also concerns over high fish intake during pregnancy due to mercury levels, which is discussed in more detail on page 75.

Although taking an omega-3 supplement is often recommended, this should not replace eating fish. Fish contains other benefits, such as iodine and protein, both of which are also important for a healthy pregnancy.

WHERE TO FIND DHA AND EPA

- Salmon (2 g per 100 g/3½ oz portion)
- Mackerel (2.6 g per 100 g/3½ oz portion)
- Fresh tuna (2.43 g per 100 g/3½ oz portion)
- Sardines (355 mg per 2 sardines)
- Trout (812 mg per 100 g/3½ oz portion)

WHERE TO FIND ALA

- Flaxseed (3.8 g per tablespoon of ground seeds) and flaxseed oil (8 g per tablespoon)
- Sunflower seeds and oil (21 mg per 25 g/1 oz)
- Rapeseed oil (1.6 g per tablespoon)
- Walnuts (2.5 g per 25 g/1 oz)

COOKING WITH OILS

Oils can be damaged so you need to take care when storing and cooking with them. Heat and light can change their chemical structure, rendering them 'rancid', which will provide less health-promoting 'free radicals'. To avoid this, use cold-pressed nut or seed oils or extra-virgin olive oil. Store them away from sunlight in a darkened cupboard and don't heat them. For this reason cooking with monounsaturated fats, such as coconut oil or a small amount of butter is recommended, as they are more stable in heat. In general, keep cooking with fats to a minimum when frying; bake, grill or slow roast instead.

GETTING THE BALANCE RIGHT

To achieve a healthy balance of macronutrients during pregnancy, aim for a plate that looks like this:

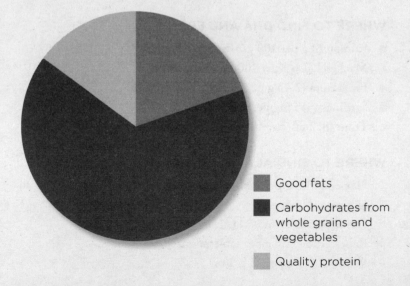

Good fats

Carbohydrates from whole grains and vegetables

Quality protein

. . .

Although it is always important to eat a balanced diet, pregnancy is one of those times in your life when you especially need to understand the building blocks of nutrition. These are, after all, the components with which you are building your child! You need to ensure that you are getting the nutrients through your diet that your body does not naturally produce – protein to build tissue and fatty acids for brain development, for example. By understanding macronutrients and micronutrients, and what they do, it is clear to see that a balanced and nutritious diet goes far beyond eating more fruit and vegetables. Everything we eat has a purpose – nutrition begins to make sense for your good health and the healthy development of your unborn child.

CHAPTER 5

MICRONUTRIENTS: THE BUILDING BLOCKS OF YOUR DIET

Good nutrition is essential for well-being throughout your whole life, but during pregnancy it plays a specific and vital role in every aspect of your baby's development. By eating a varied and wholesome diet you will be giving your baby a very healthy start in life. In this chapter we will look at the specific vitamins and minerals that you and your developing baby need throughout each trimester of pregnancy.

ESSENTIAL NUTRITION

As your baby develops with each trimester so does the importance of certain micronutrients, also called vitamins and minerals. During very early pregnancy, for example, folic acid is vital for the healthy development of your baby's spine; during the second trimester vitamin D supports the development of the skeleton; during the last trimester it is important to build up stores of iron in preparation for labour. So although a balanced diet of macronutrients (see Chapter 4) and micronutrients are needed throughout pregnancy, it is important to ensure that particular nutritional deficiencies do not occur at specific stages of pregnancy. Your body can manufacture some of the nutrients that you and your baby will need during the pregnancy, but many of them need to come from your diet.

Nutrients can be split into vitamins and minerals, and there are 13 different vitamins essential to your health. Many nutrients work in synergy – vitamin C, for example, supports the absorption of iron from food, and vitamin D the absorption of calcium. Once again balance is key to good nutrition; like food groups, vitamins do not work in isolation. These essential vitamins can be separated into fat-soluble vitamins A, D, E and K that can be stored by your body, and water-soluble vitamins C and B-complex, which are not stored in the body for very long. Water-soluble vitamins need to be consumed in your diet on a regular basis to get the right levels needed for a healthy pregnancy.

What to eat to obtain the essential vitamins and in what quantity can be daunting, but getting the correct amount of vitamin B12, for example, can be as easy as eating a yoghurt daily. Once you are aware of the levels needed and how to achieve them it is simply a case of making the right food choices.

RECOMMENDED AMOUNTS

Everyone has a different need for a nutrient depending on age, gender, weight and level of activity. Pregnant and breastfeeding women have been categorised as groups with a greater need for particular nutrients than others. An 'average' amount of each nutrient needed during these times is determined by measuring how much is needed to keep a stable blood level of the nutrient to prevent signs of disease, and these are guidelines to be used as a minimum.

The figure that the statisticians arrive at is called the Nutrient Reference Value (NRV); this used to be called the Recommended Daily Allowance (RDA). This is the amount that is seen as sufficient for 97.5 per cent of the population. The most recent National Diet and Nutrition Survey in the UK suggests that most people are not meeting the lower reference nutrient intake (LRNI). For example, 9 out of 10 women do not get the recommended intake of iron, vitamin A, calcium, zinc, magnesium and iodine. With these vitamins being essential to health, especially during pregnancy, it is really important that you are meeting the NRV of each essential vitamin as soon as you fall pregnant, and preferably before. This chapter will look at the essential vitamins and minerals for each stage of pregnancy and how to consume the recommended amount.

VITAMIN A

Vitamin A is a fat-soluble vitamin essential to your developing baby. It is a potent antioxidant and supports the development of the immune system, even increasing immune tolerance in your baby's adult life, and the development of your baby's healthy skin and eyes.

You can get vitamin A in two forms: retinol from animal sources, and beta-carotene from plant sources. Because of its status as a fat-soluble nutrient, there has been concern about excess intake of vitamin A in the form of retinol during pregnancy. In the past, pregnant women were recommended to eat liver as a good source of iron during pregnancy. However, animal liver also contains high levels of retinol, which the body can find difficult to eliminate if there is a daily intake of more than 2,900 µg from a combination of food and supplements. You won't be able to get anywhere near this amount from eating a balanced diet and avoiding high-dose supplements so there is no need to be too concerned about this. However, because vitamin A can accumulate in body tissue, and excessive intake was associated with the increased rate of babies born with birth defects, it is important to be aware of this.

The vegetable source of vitamin A, beta-carotene, has not shown to have this effect in high amounts. This is because beta-carotene is converted by your body into components of vitamin A if and when your body needs it. Therefore eating food sources that are rich in beta-carotene is recommended and favoured during pregnancy. As with any health 'scare', it tends to result in a public fear and avoidance, swinging from one extreme to another. This arguably leaves pregnant women at a greater risk of deficiency of this vital nutrient, rather than toxicity, and consequences of vitamin A deficiency can be just as devastating.

NATURAL SOURCES OF VITAMIN A

- Eggs (110 µg per medium egg)
- Whole milk (58 µg per half pint)
- Carrots (1,000 µg per 3 tablespoons)
- Mangoes (240 µg per 2 slices)
- Fresh apricots (54 µg per 3 fruit)
- Broccoli (60 µg per 75g/2¾ oz)
- Salmon (59 µg per 100g/3½ oz)
- Sweet potatoes (1,400 µg per whole potato)

HOW MUCH VITAMIN A DO I NEED?

During pregnancy you need 700 µg per day of vitamin A and 950 µg per day when breastfeeding. A 1 µg measure of beta-carotene is the equivalent of 6 µg of retinol.

B VITAMINS

All B vitamins are important for healthy growth, including biotin, B6 and B2, but the most crucial during pregnancy are folate (vitamin B9) and vitamin B12. Because the B vitamin family work in synergy, many of the foods rich in these two important vitamins are rich sources of all the B vitamins.

FOLATE

Folate is perhaps the most widely known essential nutrient during pregnancy. It is a member of the B vitamin family and needed for the production of DNA in the developing baby's cells. Folates are water-soluble compounds that are sometimes referred to as vitamin B9. As a pregnant woman your blood supply is expanding significantly throughout the pregnancy with the production of new red blood cells, and this process requires a generous supply of folate.

Folic acid is one part of this group of folates and deficiency has been linked to a developmental abnormality in the unborn baby known as a neural tube defect (such as spina bifida), which arises between 24–28 days after conception. Supplementation during the three-month preconception period and first 12 weeks of pregnancy reduces this risk by up to 70 per cent, as well as reducing the risk of 'small for gestational age' babies, and cleft lip and palate. Studies have also suggested that the use of folate supplements around the time of conception is associated with a lower risk of autistic disorders. The Growing Up in Singapore Towards Healthy Outcomes (GUSTO) study in 2014 evaluated the health of the mother and concluded that healthy folate levels reduced the risk of antenatal depression in pregnant women. It is universally accepted that folates are vitally important for the health of your unborn baby, your future child and your own well-being.

Once pregnant, women in the UK are routinely advised to take a supplement of synthetically reproduced folic acid. Recent research, however, shows that there might be greater benefits to taking the folic acid not in isolation, but in the complete folate complex as found in food. As I mentioned previously, many nutrients work in synergy, the co-dependency of folate and vitamin B12 is a primary example of this and they rely on one another for the successful formation of genetic material (DNA) during intense periods of development, such as in pregnancy. If you are taking a pregnancy supplement, look for one that contains both vitamin B12 and folate.

Recently there has been a significant amount of interest in the body's use of naturally formed folate found in food and food-state supplements, which are chemically identical or closely resemble vitamins found in food, compared to the synthetic form of folic acid found in fortified foods and the majority of other supplements (see Chapter 7 for a more in-depth look at supplements). The two are used very differently by the body. Synthetic folic acid does not cross the placenta in the same way it does in the naturally occurring food folate form. Therefore getting as much folate from your food and through food-state supplements is important in pregnancy (see page 92).

Although synthetic folic acid does not carry all the benefits of naturally occurring folate, it has been shown to reduce neural tube defects in the early stages of pregnancy. You should still take this if you cannot eat folate-rich foods or get your hands on food-state supplements.

NATURAL SOURCES OF FOLATE

The word 'folate' comes from the Latin word 'folium' meaning leaf, which will help you remember that green leafy plants are rich sources of folate.

- All green leafy vegetables (65–85 µg per 200 g/7 oz)
- Lentils (150 µg per 65 g/2½ oz)
- Chickpeas (140 µg per 65 g/2½ oz)
- Peas (20 µg per tablespoon)
- Oranges (50 µg per large orange)
- Fortified breakfast cereals (as folic acid) (25–100 µg per 35 g/ 1½ oz depending on brand)
- Milk (15 µg per 250 ml/8½ fl oz)
- Broccoli (65–85 µg per 100 g/3½ oz)

HOW MUCH FOLATE DO I NEED?

The recommended daily intake of folate during pregnancy is 400 µg from supplements for the first 12 weeks and from eating folate-rich foods on a regular basis. During breastfeeding 260 µg daily is recommended. If you have had a previous neural tube defect in pregnancy, larger doses of up to 4 mg daily are recommended the month before conception and during the first trimester.

VITAMIN B12

Vitamin B12 is essential for the formation of healthy red blood cells and therefore a healthy blood supply. As blood supply increases during pregnancy, B12 becomes particularly important. Vitamin B12 is also needed for the development of your baby's nervous system and ability to produce energy for growth. It works very closely with folate (see page 49) and having adequate levels of both of these vitamins can reduce the risk of spina bifida in the baby. Vitamin B12 is also responsible for moderating homocysteine levels in the body. High homocysteine during pregnancy can slow the unborn baby's growth and increase the risk of miscarriage.

A special enzyme in your digestive tract called intrinsic factor, or IF, is needed for vitamin B12 absorption. Autoimmune diseases and age can affect your production of IF. This results in a condition called pernicious anaemia, which can produce symptoms such as pica (see page 65), pale skin, loss of appetite, shortness of breath and depression. This condition is more likely to occur if you are of Scandinavian or Northern European descent, or have a family history of the condition. If you are experiencing any of these symptoms and are found to be vitamin B12 deficient through a blood test, you may be advised to have regular vitamin B12 injections.

B12 deficiency is also more common if you follow a vegan diet (see page 99) as many of the foods rich in B12 are not consumed.

NATURAL SOURCES OF VITAMIN B12

- Beef (1.5 µg per 100 g/3½ oz)
- Oily fish, especially sardines (4–6 µg per 100 g/3½ oz)
- Fresh tuna (1 µg per tuna steak)
- Milk (0.9–1.2 µg per 250 ml/8½ fl oz)
- Yoghurt (1.4 µg per 120 g/4¼ oz)
- Cheese (1.1 µg per 100 g/3½ oz)

- Eggs (0.6 µg per egg)
- Yeast extract (0.6–2 µg per 4 g)

HOW MUCH VITAMIN B12 DO I NEED?

You need a minimum of 1.5 µg daily during pregnancy. This increases to 2 µg daily during breastfeeding.

CHOLINE

Although not strictly a vitamin or mineral, choline is crucial. It works with folate and the production of the chemical substance acetylcholine for healthy brain and nervous system development, which takes place from day 56 of pregnancy through to four years of age! Optimum choline during the last trimester can also protect your baby's vulnerability to stress-related illness later in life. Good sources of choline are eggs yolks, dairy products from grass-fed animals, meat from organic or grass-fed animals and fish. Women are advised to consume 450 mg daily during the last trimester of pregnancy and during breastfeeding (this is 25 mg more than non-pregnant women).

VITAMIN C

An antioxidant is a type of nutrient that has the ability to protect cells against damage from daily wear and tear. Vitamin C is an important antioxidant during pregnancy. It supports the growth and repair of new tissue, including bones, teeth and skin. In addition, it is important for wound healing and for fighting off infection, so is a useful nutrient after the birth, and it supports iron absorption from food.

NATURAL SOURCES OF VITAMIN C

Remember that the riper the fruit, the richer its nutrients:

- Green leafy vegetables (approx. 80 mg per 100 g/3½ oz)
- Strawberries (in season) (62 mg per 7 fruits)

A WORD ON FRUIT

The sugar found in fruit is known as fructose. Fructose is metabolised differently in the body. Glucose can be metabolised by all cells in the body, but fructose can only be metabolised by the liver if we eat it in significant amounts, such as in a high consumption of fruit juices. When your fructose consumption is too much for the liver, it starts turning it into fat. Throughout evolutionary history we have only eaten fruit in small quantities, when in season and ripe. However, food manufacturers are using more fructose syrup to sweeten foods and drinks in a bid to make them seem 'healthier'.

Many experts such as Professor Lustig, a paediatric endocrinologist, claim that fructose is in fact the real danger in our modern diets. One of the reasons for this is that it can affect your body's use of the hormone leptin, which controls fat metabolism and can therefore lead to easy weight gain. This may be true to a degree, but it is important to remember that this is when fructose has been extracted and isolated by food manufacturers and not when it is found naturally within the whole fruit. When in fruit, fructose is combined with fibre and this dramatically changes the way the liver deals with it. Don't stop eating fruit, as it is an excellent source of nutrients, but just be aware of fruit juices where the pulp has been removed and foods that have added fructose.

- Broccoli (51 mg per 30 g/1 oz)
- New potatoes (with skins on) (13–20 mg per 100 g/3½ oz)
- Frozen peas (22 mg per 100 g/3½ oz)
- Blackcurrants (181 mg per 100 g/3½ oz)
- Oranges and fresh orange juice (not from concentrate) (54 mg per orange)
- Sweet potatoes (with skins on) (19 mg per 100 g/3½ oz)
- Kiwi fruit (64 mg per fruit)
- Tomatoes (raw) (12.7 mg per 100 g/3½ oz)
- Red peppers (raw) (95 mg per 75 g/3½ oz)
- Cranberries (13.3 mg per 100 g/3½ oz)

HOW MUCH VITAMIN C DO I NEED?

50 mg a day during pregnancy is recommended, increasing to 70 mg a day during breastfeeding.

VITAMIN D

Vitamin D helps with the absorption of calcium and phosphorous for building healthy, strong bones for you and your baby. The second trimester is a crucial time for the development of your baby's skeleton, so vitamin D and minerals such as calcium are of particular importance in this trimester. It also stimulates the growth of collagen and cartilage in your baby's joints and immune cells. Recent research has shown that vitamin D plays a direct role in learning, memory and mood; another important aspect for your developing baby and your postnatal health. An adequate intake of vitamin D during pregnancy is associated with strong bones and reduces the risk of rickets, poor teeth formation and osteoporosis in later life. Adequate vitamin D is also associated with less suscep-tibility to antenatal and postnatal depression.

Vitamin D is actually a collective term for many types of vitamin D, including the better known D2 and D3. Plant-derived vitamin

D2 is thought to be less effective at maintaining blood levels of vitamin D than the vitamin D3 form made from a diet that contains animal products. Vitamin D3 can also be synthesised in your skin through UVB (ultraviolet B) sunlight. However, the strength of the UVB light is not strong enough in the UK in autumn and winter to provide sufficient levels. Additionally, the fact that many people now use sunscreens and spend lots of time indoors, in office-bound jobs and for leisure, has further limited exposure to this important vitamin. The darker your skin, the harder it is to generate vitamin D, i.e. you need greater amounts of UVB sunlight. Low levels of sunshine in the UK and a reduction in vitamin D-rich food (such as eggs and liver) during pregnancy mean that it is advisable to supplement with vitamin D during the winter months.

National Diet and Nutrition Surveys (NDNS) in the UK have shown that around 70 per cent of women are deficient in vitamin D. Rickets, once thought to be caused by poverty or malnutrition, is now coming back, and more pregnant and breastfeeding women are deficient. An adequate intake of vitamin D during pregnancy has also been associated with a reduced risk of pre-eclampsia (see page 118), and wheezing in children up to aged two.

Vitamin D works alongside magnesium, calcium, manganese and phosphorous in supporting bone formation in the unborn baby. Many of these minerals are also found in vitamin D-rich foods.

NATURAL SOURCES OF VITAMIN D
- Mackerel (9 g per 100 g/3½ oz)
- Sardines (10.13 µg per 100 g/3½ oz)
- Salmon (11.2 µg per 100 g/3½ oz)
- Eggs (1.02 µg per large egg)
- Beef (1.05 µg per 100 g/3½ oz)
- Tofu (3.9 µg per 100 g/3½ oz)
- Mushrooms (such as shiitake or oyster) (7.5–10 µg per 100 g/3½ oz)
- Dairy products (such as whole milk) (2–3.1 µg per 250 ml)

HOW MUCH VITAMIN D DO I NEED?

Consuming 10 µg of vitamin D a day is recommended during pregnancy and breastfeeding, especially in those women pregnant between October to April.

VITAMIN E

Vitamin E has a powerful antioxidant action, helping to protect your cells and those of your baby against damage from daily wear and tear. It can also protect your baby from developing asthma and allergies later in life. Again, there is a significant difference between synthetic vitamin E and that found in nature, and this is explained in Chapter 7 on supplements.

NATURAL SOURCES OF VITAMIN E

- Avocados (2.1 mg per 100 g/3½ oz)
- Grass-fed or organic meat (0.4 mg per 100g/3½ oz) – grass-fed animal fats are estimated to be four times higher in vitamin E than those of grain-fed animals
- Sunflower seeds (33.3 mg per 100g/3½ oz)
- Butter (2.3 mg per 100g/3½ oz)
- Almonds (26.2 mg per 100 g/3½ oz)
- Hazelnuts (15 mg per 100 g/3½ oz)

HOW MUCH VITAMIN E DO I NEED?

Approximately 4–5 mg a day during pregnancy and breastfeeding appears to be sufficient for most women. If you have a diet rich in polyunsaturated fats (see page 41), you may require a little more as vitamin E is used to process these fats in the body.

VITAMIN K

Vitamin K helps to lay down calcium in the bones and is needed for normal blood clotting. There are three forms of vitamin K: K1, K2 and K3. Vitamin K2 is transported across the placenta at a higher rate than vitamin K1, to support healthy blood clotting in babies once they are born.

Some newborns are born with insufficient vitamin K levels and therefore are at risk of haemorrhagic disease of the newborn (HDN) especially if they are pre-term or of low birth weight. Vitamin K2 injections or drops are routinely given to newborns, but you do have the right to refuse this. By day eight your baby's own ability to produce clotting factors is at its peak, especially if your pregnancy diet has been healthy.

NATURAL SOURCES OF VITAMIN K2

- Fermented foods such as sauerkraut (13 µg per 100 g/3½ oz) – see page 206 for recipe
- Grass-fed animal fats found in butter and cheese (7 µg per 100 g/ 3½ oz)
- All green leafy vegetables, but especially kale (817 µg per 100 g/ 3½ oz)
- Broccoli (102 µg per 100 g/3½ oz)
- Sprouts, such as alfalfa sprouts (30.5 µg per 100 g/3½ oz)

HOW MUCH VITAMIN K DO I NEED?

There is no recommended dose for vitamin K and taking supplements isn't necessary if you are eating plenty of the above foods in your daily diet. Healthy bacteria in the gut is involved in producing vitamin K and therefore it is important to optimise your levels of this.

ZINC

The mineral zinc supports cell division, which is extremely rapid in the early stages of pregnancy. It is needed to make healthy white blood cells for your baby's immune system and nervous system, and supports the digestion of fats, proteins and carbohydrates for both of you. It is also needed for wound healing and growth. Zinc is a vital nutrient for the stability of hormones, including oestrogen and progesterone. Zinc deficiency can block folate absorption so taking in zinc-rich food is very important for you and your baby. Healthy zinc levels can also support a healthy birth weight.

White spots on your nails and a poor sense of taste and smell can be indications of zinc deficiency.

NATURAL SOURCES OF ZINC

- Whole grains (2–3 mg per 100 g/3½ oz)
- All meat, especially lamb (4.7 mg per 100 g/3½ oz)
- Oysters (90 mg per 100 g/3½ oz)
- Dairy products, such as yoghurt (0.6 mg per 100 g/3½ oz)
- Pumpkin seeds (7.5 mg per 100 g/3½ oz)
- Almonds (3.1 mg per 100 g/3½ oz)
- Chickpeas (1.5 mg per 100 g/3½ oz)

HOW MUCH ZINC DO I NEED?

During pregnancy 7 mg of zinc per day is recommended. In the first four months of breastfeeding your intake needs to increase to around 13 mg and after this period drops to 9.5 mg.

IRON

Monitoring iron levels during pregnancy is important for a number of reasons. Iron is needed for the healthy brain development of your unborn baby (and during their infancy too) and it is important for building a healthy blood supply. In the third trimester, your baby will accumulate 2 mg of iron a day so that by the time he is full term he will have accumulated 150–250 mg in total, most of which will be in the form of haemoglobin, which carries oxygen around the body for you and your baby. This is why premature babies are at a greater risk of iron deficiency. This then creates a good store of iron (called ferritin) of around 60 mg. Your baby then uses this to build lean tissue for the first six months of life. After this he will become more dependent on food and milk for iron. At your baby's birth, ask your midwife to only clamp the umbilical cord once it has stopped pulsing as this can also improve your baby's storage of iron.

Healthy iron stores during pregnancy can also improve a healthy birth weight, reduce the risk of premature birth and of your baby developing asthma in later childhood years. It's pretty important! Because your body adapts during pregnancy and breastfeeding to ensure your baby naturally receives a supply of iron, recommended intakes for pregnant women are the same as those for non-pregnant women. If, however, you began your pregnancy with low iron stores, I advise that you build up your intake through supplementation and diet to support your pregnancy, especially in the last trimester.

Women are routinely screened for iron-deficiency anaemia at the beginning of their pregnancy. Signs of deficiency might include feeling dizzy and lethargic, having pale skin and being constipated. As your baby grows, however, iron demands increase and therefore I feel that women should be monitored throughout the pregnancy, especially in the last trimester when iron stores need to be high in preparation for labour.

NATURAL SOURCES OF IRON

- Spinach (2.7 mg per 100 g/3½ oz) – cook spinach rather than eating it raw as this improves iron absorption. Steaming spinach is the best method
- Chicken thigh (1.3 mg per 100 g/3½ oz)

- Grass-fed beef (2 mg per 100 g/3½ oz)
- Lentils (3.3 mg per 100 g/3½ oz)
- Eggs (0.6 mg per large egg)
- Dried apricots (2.7 mg per 100 g/3½ oz) – organic apricots are preferable as the non-organic form use sulphur dioxide as a preservative and to prevent discolouration, which can increase wind and may be problematic for those with respiratory conditions such as asthma. The use of preservatives such as sulphur dioxide is prohibited in the organic growth or production process

Iron from meat is easier to absorb than iron from plants and pulses. The darker the meat, the more iron it contains. Therefore the darker meat in poultry, such as the leg or thigh, is best for iron levels.

VITAMIN C AND IRON

Vitamin C increases the absorption of iron from food, so eating foods rich in vitamin C with your iron-rich foods can boost your iron levels.

HOW MUCH IRON DO I NEED?

During pregnancy and breastfeeding you need 14.8 mg per day. Also see page 92 on supplements.

SELENIUM

Selenium is a trace mineral that protects your cells and your baby's developing cells from wear and tear, as well as helping to build a strong immune system. It can protect against chromosome breakages, a cause of birth defects and miscarriages. Having a good intake of selenium during pregnancy can reduce your baby's risk of developing eczema and wheezing (an early sign of asthma) too.

PHYTIC ACID

Phytic acid is present in beans, seeds and grains (especially in the hull or bran). It has been shown to 'bind' to important minerals such as calcium, magnesium, zinc and iron, and to vitamin D. It can also inhibit important enzymes that digest our food. High 'phytate' diets have been associated with conditions such as osteoporosis and rickets because of how they affect calcium and vitamin D levels. Individuals with a sensitive digestion can also find these foods 'irritating', bringing on symptoms such as wind, cramping and bloating. This has meant that foods rich in phytates have been dismissed by many, which is a shame because they are packed full of goodness. The way in which the food is produced can increase or decrease phytic acid, and those foods grown using modern high-phosphate fertilisers are estimated to increase the levels in comparison to those grown in natural compost.

There are a number of ways to reduce phytic acid. Soaking grains and pulses overnight can reduce phytate content that can be problematic in some people. You can also decrease phytic acid and increase vitamins and enzymes that improve digestibility by 'sprouting' your grains or pulses. To do this you need to soak the seeds, rinse them and repeat this process until they begin to germinate or 'sprout'.

Unfortunately phytic acid is also found in cocoa products, so this includes chocolate products.

NATURAL SOURCES OF SELENIUM

- Whole grains such as wholewheat (70.7 µg per 100 g/3½ oz)
- Brazil nuts (organic preferably) (504 µg per 100 g/3½ oz)
- Fish, especially fresh tuna (92 µg per 100 g/3½ oz)
- Prawns (38 µg per 100 g/3½ oz)
- Eggs (15 µg per 100 g/3½ oz)
- Lentils (6 µg per 100 g/3½ oz)
- Red meat (28–30 µg per 100 g/3½ oz)

The selenium content of food is directly proportional to the selenium content of the soil in which it was grown. In the UK, selenium intakes have fallen with the increased use of European grains that are less rich in the mineral (see page 88).

HOW MUCH SELENIUM DO I NEED?

During pregnancy 60 µg of selenium a day is recommended and 75 µg a day during breastfeeding.

CALCIUM

Calcium is another essential nutrient for your health and that of your baby. It is needed for the development of healthy bones and teeth, a healthy nervous system, muscle contraction and blood clotting, which is particularly important during the birthing process. Over the course of the pregnancy you will be transferring around 30 g (1 oz) of calcium from your body to your baby's. Some women find that their teeth become more fragile and prone to fillings or breaking because calcium is being taken from their teeth and bones to support the developing baby.

Calcium also works very closely with other minerals such as magnesium, manganese and zinc, and vitamins B12 and D to support your baby's bone development.

CALCIUM IN DAIRY PRODUCTS

It is well known that dairy products are a rich source of calcium. However, in order for calcium to be well absorbed by your body, it requires a good ratio of magnesium too. The calcium/magnesium ratio is pretty poor in dairy products and so the calcium provision is not as good as people think. Green leafy vegetables and other plant sources of calcium provide a higher amount of magnesium and therefore a more effective calcium/magnesium ratio.

NATURAL SOURCES OF CALCIUM

- Whole milk (276 mg per 250 ml/8½ fl oz)
- Yoghurt (310–390 mg per 250 g/9 oz)
- Cottage cheese (138 mg per 200 g/7 oz)
- Fish with soft bones, such as sardines and whitebait (325 mg per 100 g/3½ oz)
- Cabbage (74 mg per 75 g/2½ oz)
- Broccoli (21 mg per 100 g/3½ oz)
- Bread (30 mg per slice)

There is also a small amount of calcium in drinking water in hard water areas.

HOW MUCH CALCIUM DO I NEED?

During pregnancy 700 mg of calcium per day is recommended, increasing to 1,250 mg per day during breastfeeding. Because of the partnership relationship with vitamin D, it is really important to increase your vitamin D intake too (see page 55).

PICA

Pica is a recurrent craving or pattern of eating non-food materials – coal or paper, for example – that lasts for at least one month. It can be more common in pregnancy and in some cases can indicate a lack of certain nutrients. Iron, zinc and vitamin B12 deficiencies are thought to be the most common triggers. Cravings can occur for the following:

- Clay
- Soil
- Ice
- Paint
- Paper
- Sand
- Coal

If you experience pica, seek support from your midwife or GP.

IODINE

Deficiency in iodine is worldwide and became the subject of the recent World Health Organisation (WHO) Technical Consultation to prevent and control iodine deficiency in pregnant and breastfeeding women, and in children under two years of age. Iodine is needed for the early stages of your baby's growth and nervous system development, especially during the first three months. Deficiency is rare in European countries but women with marginal iodine levels prior to becoming pregnant can start to show signs of deficiency during pregnancy.

Healthy iodine intake can improve your baby's protection against disease for life, as well as improving IQ – it's worth eating a few eggs for! I recommend taking a pregnancy multinutrient that contains iodine. Obvious signs of deficiency are a goitre on the neck, which is a large swelling or nodule. If this occurs visit your GP.

NATURAL SOURCES OF IODINE

- Eggs (24 μg per large egg)
- Cod (99 μg per 100 g/3½ oz)
- Seafood (35 μg per 100 g/3½ oz)
- Seaweeds (16–500 μg per 500 mg) – examples include dulse, kombu, nori, arame and wakame

A sea green culinary ingredient is an excellent source of iodine and can be added on to food as a seasoning.

HOW MUCH IODINE DO I NEED?

For pregnant and breastfeeding women, 250 μg iodine per day is recommended.

MAGNESIUM

Although not a 'core' nutrient during pregnancy, it is magnesium that 'fixes' calcium into the bones. It is also used for muscle contractions (important during labour) and regulates blood pressure. Seventy per cent of Western women are estimated to be deficient in magnesium, and healthy levels of this mineral may reduce the risk of pre-eclampsia (see page 118) and associated high blood pressure during pregnancy.

NATURAL SOURCES OF MAGNESIUM

- Green leafy vegetables, especially spinach and Swiss chard (78 mg per 100 g/3½ oz)
- All nuts, especially cashew nuts (74 mg per 25 g/1 oz)
- Black beans, edamame beans and kidney beans (40–60 mg per 75 g/2½ oz)

- Avocados (44 mg per 150 g/5 oz)
- Bananas (32 mg per medium-sized banana)
- Quinoa (45 mg per 50 g/2 oz)

HOW MUCH MAGNESIUM DO I NEED?

There is no increased need for magnesium during pregnancy, but as many women are estimated to be deficient it is important to make sure you have it in your prenatal supplement (see page 10). The current recommended dose for women is 375 mg per day.

GETTING THE BALANCE RIGHT

Nutrition is a wonderful and complex science, and understanding how the macro and micro factors work to develop and nurture you and your unborn child is powerful knowledge indeed. Research on the matter is vast and sometimes it can be difficult to take on board all of the things you have read and heard on nutrition, especially when new research is emerging all of the time. One thing remains consistent – that eating a balanced diet is beneficial to health, starting as early as possible before you conceive. Vitamins work in synergy, so eating a good variety of foods will give you the optimum access to all the nutrients you need. The use of supplements may lay the focus on individual vitamins in isolation, but in a natural state they exist as part of a food complex. Eggs, for example, contain vitamins A, D, B2, B12 and folates; cauliflower contains vitamin C, K and folates, and so a variety of foods eaten in combination will provide you with your daily recommended dose. By seeing vitamins less as separate entities and more as the building blocks of the meals you create, it will become easier to provide yourself and your unborn child with all the nutrients you need for good health. Supplements have their place, as we will discover in Chapter 7, but eating a fresh, varied and colourful diet is the healthier, more enjoyable way to increase your vitamin intake.

NUTRIENTS KNOW-HOW AT A GLANCE

We've covered a lot of ground in this chapter so here is a quick-reference chart to help you navigate which nutrients you need and when.

Nutrient	How much do I need daily?	Is there a time I need it more than most?	Which are some of the best sources?
Vitamin A	700 µg when pregnant; 950 µg when breastfeeding	Breastfeeding	Broccoli, whole milk, eggs, fresh apricots, salmon
Folate	400 µg when pregnant; 260 µg when breastfeeding	Pre conception First trimester Breastfeeding	Pulses, green leafy vegetables, lentils, peas, broccoli
Vitamin B12	1.5 µg when pregnant; 2 µg when breastfeeding	Breastfeeding	Yoghurt, milk, eggs, oily fish, yeast extract
Choline	450 mg	Third trimester Breastfeeding	Egg yolks, grass-fed or organic meat and dairy
Vitamin C	50 mg per day; 70 mg when breastfeeding	Breastfeeding	Green leafy vegetables, strawberries, broccoli, blackcurrants, red peppers

Nutrient	How much do I need daily?	Is there a time I need it more than most?	Which are some of the best sources?
Vitamin D	10 µg	Second trimester	Oily fish, eggs, dairy products
Vitamin E	4–5 mg		Avocados, grass-fed meat, almonds, sunflower seeds
Vitamin K	No recommended dose	Breastfeeding	Fermented foods, broccoli, alfalfa sprouts
Zinc	7 mg during pregnancy; 9.5–13 mg during breastfeeding	Breastfeeding	Seafood, whole grains, dairy products, pumpkin seeds, nuts, pulses
Iron	14.8 mg	Third trimester Breastfeeding	Lentils, eggs, dried apricots, green leafy vegetables, meat
Selenium	60 µg during pregnancy; 75 µg during breastfeeding	Breastfeeding	Whole grains, fish, eggs, brazil nuts, meat
Calcium	700 mg during pregnancy; 1,250 mg during breastfeeding	Second trimester Breastfeeding	Dairy products, cabbage, broccoli, bread

Nutrient	How much do I need daily?	Is there a time I need it more than most?	Which are some of the best sources?
Magnesium	375 mg	Throughout pregnancy	Avocados, cashew nuts, green leafy vegetables, kidney beans
Iodine	250 mg	Throughout pregnancy Breastfeeding	Eggs, seafood, iodised salt, seaweeds

CHAPTER 6

FOODS TO AVOID DURING PREGNANCY

Hormonal changes during pregnancy can weaken the immune system and make you more susceptible to infections, especially if you are not eating a healthy and nutritious diet. In this chapter I will advise you on which foods to avoid and why, and provide helpful and nutritious substitutes. Official guidelines may vary from one pregnancy to the next, and from country to country, but the correct and hygienic way to treat food is a universal constant. I will explain how to prepare and store foods to minimise your exposure to infection, and also give you tips on eating out and the importance of reading labels.

In the section that follows, you will find details of the foods that the Department of Health currently recommends avoiding during pregnancy. Your midwife will also give you a booklet that includes the current guidelines.

CHEESE

Do not eat:

- **Soft blue-veined cheese.** Mould-ripened blue cheese, such as Gorgonzola, Danish blue and Roquefort. These can contain listeria bacteria and cause listeriosis, an infection that affects the unborn baby. It is not harmful to eat hard blue cheeses, such as Stilton.
- **Rinded soft cheeses.** These are Brie, Camembert and goat's cheese (also called chèvre) with a similar mould rind. These may also contain listeria bacteria.

CAN I EAT COOKED BRIE AND BLUE CHEESE DURING PREGNANCY?

Yes, soft goat's cheese, Brie, Camembert and blue cheeses are fine to eat when cooked, but make sure they are cooked all the way through. This destroys any listeria bacteria that might be present.

It is safe to eat:

- Cheddar
- Edam
- Emmental
- Gouda
- Gruyère
- Jarlsberg
- Parmesan
- Stilton
- Grana padano
- Cottage cheese
- Mozzarella
- Feta
- Cream cheese
- Paneer
- Ricotta
- Halloumi
- Hard goat's cheese

MILK PRODUCTS

Avoid all unpasteurised milk products. This includes cream, milk and cheese from cows, goats and sheep.

Good alternatives: All pasteurised dairy products are fine (with the exception of soft rind cheese – see page 71). Crème fraîche, mascarpone, ricotta and fromage frais are fine too. Alternatives to dairy are nut milk, such as almond and cashew milks, or hemp, rice and oat milks. They are lighter and help to bring variety and reduce your consumption of dairy if this is a problem for you.

EGGS

Be careful of raw, undercooked or soft-boiled eggs, and any foods that contain these such as home-made mayonnaise, hollandaise sauce, some meringues, mousses and some custards and ice creams. This is because of the risk of salmonella, although this risk is now deemed to be less than previously thought. To reduce the risk of salmonella, make sure that eggs are thoroughly cooked until the whites and yolks are solid.

Good alternatives: You can use natural egg replacers for home-made mayonnaise or custards (see page 215). Choose non-egg puddings such as sorbet or my recipe for Blueberry Ice Cream (see page 209).

PÂTÉ

Don't eat pâté, including vegetable pâtés, as these are also thought to be a potential source of listeria.

Good alternatives: Choose dips instead, such as the delicious Creamy Spinach Dip (see page 202).

MEAT

It is not advisable to eat raw or even undercooked meat during pregnancy because it is a potential source of the parasite Toxoplasma gondii, causing the infection toxoplasmosis. In a healthy adult and child, the immune system is strong enough to prevent the parasite causing serious illness, but pregnant women are more vulnerable. Raw meat can also be a source of E. coli and salmonella bacteria.

Cook all meat, especially pork and poultry, so that there is no trace of pink or blood when you cut the meat. The Food Standards

Agency (FSA) has recently changed the advice for pregnant women, recommending that they also exercise caution with cold cured meats including salami, chorizo, pepperoni and Parma ham.

Tip: You can reduce the risk of parasitic infection by freezing cured or fermented meats for four days before you eat them. Always make sure you defrost them thoroughly before eating.

LIVER

Avoid eating liver and liver products, such as pâté or liver sausage. These can be a source of undercooked meat but also contain a lot of vitamin A, which is thought to have adverse effects on your baby's growth if consumed in very high amounts (see page 48).

Good alternatives: See 5-Minute Mackerel Pâté (see page 204) and Beetroot and Hazelnut Dip (see page 201).

RAW OR UNDERCOOKED FISH

It is not harmful to eat raw or lightly cooked fish, such as some sushi dishes, but you need to ensure that the fish, preferably wild, has been frozen beforehand. This information should be on the packaging. The freezing process kills any unwanted bacteria on the fish. If you are in doubt, don't eat it. You can also contact the FSA for advice (see page 214).

Good alternatives: Canned fish (preferably in natural spring water or olive oil as these are healthier than the brine options), vegetarian sushi and teriyaki dishes.

FISH

Pregnant and breastfeeding women are advised by the Department of Health to be mindful of eating certain fish. They are advised to avoid consuming shark, swordfish and marlin because of their potential high levels of mercury (see box, page 76), which can affect an unborn baby's developing nervous system. Mercury has also been associated with an increased risk of postnatal depression (see page 132).

It is also recommended that you be mindful of how much oily fish you eat. Oily fish include fresh tuna (not canned), salmon, trout, mackerel, herring, sardines and pilchards. This is because 'fattier' fish, such as tuna or salmon, can be a potential source of mercury and other pollutants, such as dioxins and polychlorinated biphenyls (PCBs). The official recommendation is that you eat no more than two portions of oily fish per week. However, I cannot stress enough how important it is *not* to avoid eating fish completely during pregnancy. There are experts that argue that the risk of avoiding fish completely during pregnancy outweighs the risk of consuming too much oily fish. Fish is an excellent source of iodine, protein, essential fatty acids and other micronutrients that are essential for the healthy growth of your unborn baby, and a moderate fish intake during pregnancy is associated with lower risk of pre-term birth and a small yet significant increase in birth weight.

There are some types of white fish that are also regarded as having similar levels of PCBs and dioxins as oily fish and therefore the same limits are recommended. These are dogfish, sea bass, sea bream, turbot, halibut and crab.

Good alternatives: You do not need to limit or avoid other types of white and non-oily fish such as cod, haddock, plaice, dab, pollock, coley, skate, hake, flounder and gurnard.

Tip: Look for oily fish that is wild or organic, rather than farmed fish. Where the fish is caught can also reduce or increase risk. The Marine Conservation Society (see page 214) is an excellent resource for checking which fish to look for.

MERCURY

Mercury belongs to a group of metals called metalloestrogens. These are known as lipophilic, which simply means fat-loving, and are therefore easily stored in human body fat. This is also a protective mechanism by the body to keep the metals away from the vital organs and growing baby. However, it is possible for some to remain in circulation and interact with the normal functioning of your brain, nervous system and immune system. Therefore the FSA recommends that pregnant women avoid eating shark, swordfish and marlin, as these fish have been found to contain higher levels of mercury. Tuna contains lower levels of mercury and therefore it is suggested that two portions of fresh tuna (i.e. two fresh tuna steaks) or four 200 g/7 oz of canned tuna a week are fine and have health benefits for the developing baby.

NUTS

Nuts are a nutritious food. They are a rich source of omega-3 fatty acids and many minerals, such as zinc and magnesium. There has been a lot of controversy over nuts in the last few years. In the past it has been recommended that pregnant and breastfeeding women avoid eating nuts, peanuts in particular, for fear that it might increase the chances of the baby developing a nut allergy.

In 2009, the government changed this advice based on new evidence published by the *Journal of the American Medical Association*, that a growing baby's exposure to nuts via the pregnant mother's diet can actually help to develop a natural tolerance to nuts. However, it is still advised that you avoid consuming nuts if there is a strong family history (i.e. with you or your partner) of nut allergies.

FOOD SAFETY

Here are some simple tips for safe preparation, cooking and storage of food:

- Check 'sell by' and 'use by' dates, and don't eat food beyond those dates.
- Take food from the back of the shelf in the supermarket as this often has the freshest produce and the later 'use by' date.
- Do not buy food if the packaging has been torn or opened.
- Unpack and put away your refrigerated and frozen foods immediately once you are home.
- Keep raw and cooked foods separately in the fridge, and ensure no juices from meat can leak into other fresh produce in the fridge.
- Always make sure raw meat is wrapped well and preferably kept at the bottom of the fridge.
- If you are saving leftovers, cover them as soon as they are cooled and refrigerate or freeze immediately. If you are refrigerating them, eat within 24 hours.
- Never re-heat food more than once. This is especially true for meat and grains.
- When preparing food, keep raw meat on a separate chopping board and use a separate knife. Never leave meat out for long periods of time, especially in the warmer summer months.
- Be careful of eating barbecued meat as it is often undercooked.

- Preferably use loose-leaf salad rather than pre-packaged salad bags as there is a small risk of listeria bacteria in these. They are often washed in unnecessary chemicals.
- Cook all meat, poultry, fish, game and egg thoroughly.
- Wash your hands thoroughly after cooking with meat. A good kitchen hand-soap is one that contains natural antimicrobial tea-tree.
- Wash all vegetables carefully, especially if you are using produce from your garden. Keep nets over vegetable patches to keep cats away (cat faeces is a source of Toxoplasma gondii).
- Make sure your fridge is below 5°C and your freezer below 18°C.

WHAT ABOUT EATING OUT?

It is obviously much harder to be 100 per cent sure of hygiene standards, so when you are eating out or getting a takeaway, choose places that you trust. If you get a takeaway and the food is not piping or steaming hot, put it in the oven to reheat until it's bubbling or steaming. Don't be afraid to ask what ingredients are in your dish when ordering in a restaurant, too. Much better to ask than to be worrying!

CAFFEINE

Consuming caffeine in large quantities has been associated with miscarriage and reduced birth weight, so limiting your intake of caffeine during pregnancy is advised.

Caffeine can be found in coffee and in all teas (other than decaffeinated – see box, page 79), such as green tea, oolong tea and black tea. It is also found in chocolate, cola drinks (including diet versions), energy drinks and some medication (especially cold and flu remedies).

Consuming up to 200 mg of caffeine per day is regarded as safe (this is the equivalent of just over two cups of instant coffee). Consuming more than 200 mg of caffeine per day may adversely affect your unborn baby, so it is advisable to consume as little as possible. I recommend that you avoid consuming caffeine completely during pregnancy, especially in the first trimester when the risk of miscarriage is higher. Also your baby does not have the liver enzymes that we accrue as adults to break down caffeine. Additionally, compounds called tannins found in many caffeine-containing drinks can also inhibit the absorption of important minerals such as iron, calcium and zinc. Caffeine is a diuretic, causing the body to expel water from the body at a faster rate and therefore it increases the risk of dehydration. It also disrupts blood-sugar management, which is very important to look after during pregnancy and breastfeeding.

Good alternatives: Redbush tea, chicory or barley coffee, and herbal teas such as fennel, peppermint, spiced chai or chamomile.

WHAT ABOUT DECAFFEINATED TEA AND COFFEE?

Legally decaffeinated coffee or tea needs to have 97 per cent of the caffeine removed to be classified as decaffeinated. This means that decaffeinated is not the same as caffeine-free, and often there will still be traces of caffeine in the product. It will also still contain the stimulating chemical theobromine, although this has not been shown to have negative consequences on the unborn baby's growth in the same way as caffeine. The decaffeination process also removes many of the beneficial antioxidants found in the cocoa bean and often involves the use of solvents. The answer is to moderate your intake of decaffeinated drinks too – try other alternative caffeine-free drinks (see above).

HOW MUCH CAFFEINE?

Chocolate	Caffeine content (mg)
50 g/2 oz plain dark chocolate	up to 50
50 g/2 oz milk chocolate	25
1 cup (280 ml) of drinking chocolate	1–8

Coffee	
1 cup (280 ml) of filter	100–115
1 cup (280 ml) of instant	75
1 mug (350 ml) of instant	100
1 single espresso	75–100
1 regular cappuccino or latte	100–200
1 regular Americano	225–300
1 cup (280 ml) of decaffeinated	4

Cola	
330 ml (11 fl oz) regular or diet	40

Energy drink	up to 80
(Containing caffeine or guarana)	

Tea	
1 cup (280 ml) from teabags or loose tea leaves	50

A word of caution: The amount of caffeine depends on the strength of the tea leaves and coffee beans used. Remember too that many coffee houses these days serve coffees with two or even three shots, depending on the cup size. The average 'shot' provides approximately 100 mg of caffeine.

ALCOHOL

There is evidence to suggest that relatively small amounts of alcohol can increase the risk of miscarriage and therefore the Department of Health recommend that pregnant women avoid drinking alcohol in the first trimester.

I GOT DRUNK BEFORE I KNEW I WAS PREGNANT

If you drank a lot of alcohol before you knew you were pregnant, try not to worry. There is nothing that you can do to change it and there is very little chance it would have caused any harm to your baby. The most important thing is that you are vigilant about your intake from the time you find out.

There is still a great deal of uncertainty about how much alcohol is safe to drink in pregnancy and therefore I suggest that you continue to avoid drinking alcohol throughout your pregnancy. This is because, aside from the concerns over the effect alcohol itself has on your growing baby, it has adverse health effects. It is a diuretic, it disrupts blood-sugar management and it reduces stores of nutrients, especially B vitamins, including folate and vitamin B12. However, if you choose to have the odd drink during pregnancy there is no evidence to suggest that one or two units (see box, page 82) a week will cause any harm to your baby.

Good alternatives: Crushed fresh mint leaves with naturally sparkling water; fresh lemon, lime or grated fresh ginger in sparkling water; 25 ml/1 fl oz of fresh fruit juice (not from concentrate) in water.

WHAT IS A UNIT OF ALCOHOL?

- 125 ml (4 fl oz) small glass of red/white/rose wine – 1.5 units
- 175 ml (6 fl oz) medium glass of red/white/rose wine – 2.1 units
- 600 ml (1 pint) of 3.6% ABV beer – 2 units
- 330 ml (11 fl oz) bottle cider or beer – 1.7 units
- 25 ml (1 fl oz) measure of gin/vodka – 1 unit

FOOD ADDITIVES

Eating fresh and home-cooked food naturally reduces your intake of unwanted additives or sugars, but packaged and processed foods may also creep into your diet from time to time. There are some additives that can be found in packaged foods that should be avoided as they are thought to have adverse effects on the growing baby when consumed in high amounts. Look out for the following on food labels:

- **Sodium benzoate.** Also known as E211, this is used in a lot of baked goods, such as cakes, biscuits, pastries, and also ice lollies and soft drinks. It too has been linked to birth abnormalities when consumed in high amounts.
- **Sulphur dioxide**. Also known as E220, this is commonly used in crisps and other potato-based snacks and in non-organic dried fruit. In animal studies, a high intake of this is associated with DNA damage.
- **Quinoline yellow and sunset yellow.** Also known as E104 and E110, these additives are often used in ice creams and desserts and, as their names suggest, give a yellow colouring to the food. They have also been associated with DNA damage.

- **Aspartame.** Also known as E951, this is a very common artificial sweetener in foods and drinks, especially diet products. It crosses the placenta easily and high intakes have been associated with birth defects and damage to the unborn baby's brain. Recently researchers have discovered the use of artificial sweeteners can disrupt glucose metabolism in a similar way to sugar.
- **Saccharine.** Also known as E954, this additive is widely used and has been associated with DNA damage in animal studies. The implications on human health are not known.

ORGANIC FOOD

Ideally the food that you eat should be as free as possible from pesticides and herbicides. Taking this into account, food produced organically is the healthier choice. It is also naturally free from genetically modified (GM) products and has lower levels of food additives. Some pesticides can contain traces of metalloproteins, including cadmium and mercury, which have been associated with reduced growth of the unborn baby and, more recently, increased risk of your baby developing obesity and Type 2 diabetes in later life. Male babies appear to be at greater risk than female.

Other studies have demonstrated that eating organic food can improve cognitive development, but these studies are far from conclusive.

Many of the chemicals used in food production (although not all!) are proven to be safe to use for public consumption below strict levels, but we don't know what happens when we consume a cocktail of these chemicals, and this is the most likely way we eat them in our modern diets.

Animals reared to produce meat and dairy are often exposed to significant amounts of antibiotics and growth hormones. Many of these are lipophilic, meaning that they remain in the fat content of the meat and the dairy products they produce. It is also argued that this routine use of medication can also be causing antibiotic resistance in animals, rendering the meat more susceptible to the bacteria campylobacter, which we then consume when we eat the meat. Animals reared to produce organic meat have strict restrictions on the amount of medication and the type of feed they are given, thus reducing the amount of exposure to these unwanted chemicals.

WHAT IS GRASS-FED MEAT?

Grass-fed meat comes from animals that eat mainly grass (as opposed to non-organic or animals that are mostly corn or soy fed). The 'rearing' method of grass-fed animals has been shown to increase the nutrient and omega-3 fatty acid content of the meat. It also provides higher levels of CLA, another fatty acid needed for healthy development of the unborn baby. Conversely, non-grass fed or non-organic meat is fed mostly on corn or soy and has a higher balance of omega-6 than omega-3.

Aside from the naturally lower levels of additives and chemicals found in organic produce, it is also believed to be more nutrient dense than non-organic, in certain food groups.

A recent review of 343 studies, which was published in the *British Journal of Nutrition*, found that organic foods are healthier than conventionally grown foods. This is primarily due to the higher levels of protective antioxidants found in these foods (shown to be around up to 69 per cent more). Organic foods were also shown to have approximately 48 per cent lower concentrations of the toxic metal cadmium.

Choosing organic can be expensive and so I recommend that you prioritise meats, dairy and rice, and choose grass-fed or organic meat. Some fruit and vegetables are grown with more pesticides than others, and the Environmental Working Group (EWG) has created a list of the 'dirty dozen' – those foods with the highest pesticide and insecticide load to help you prioritise your weekly shop.

The 'Dirty Dozen' foods are:

- Apples
- Celery
- Cherry tomatoes
- Cucumbers
- Grapes
- Nectarines
- Peaches
- Potatoes
- Snap peas
- Spinach
- Strawberries
- Sweet bell peppers

plus

- Chilli peppers
- Kale/collard greens

The above non-organic fruit and vegetables can be peeled or scrubbed to remove traces of pesticides, but remember that much of the nutritional content exists just below the surface of the peel. Look for certification of organic status from one of the Department for Environment, Food & Rural Affairs (DEFRA) approved Organic Control bodies.

IS SOYA SAFE?

It is often assumed that meat and dairy alternatives are the healthier option, but this is not always the case.

One of the most popular meat substitutes, soya, contains a group of plant chemicals called phytoestrogens. These compounds can have a similar, albeit weak, effect on the body's level of the hormone oestrogen. Some theories suggest that eating these phytoestrogens during pregnancy can affect the fertility and sexual health of the baby, but these claims are not well founded. Phytoestrogens often come as a 'team' within food and include genistein, daidzein and isoflavone, but many of the studies on phytoestrogens use only one of these, for example just genistein on its own. This increases its 'oestrogenic' effect and brings with it health concerns when on its own in high doses – doses that would be hard to reach from eating whole soya foods such as tempeh.

Therefore my advice is to make sure that when you do consume soya, you consume it in its whole form and preferably fermented (research into soya products that has shown soya to be supportive to health have studied cultures where fermented soya has the highest consumption) such as tofu, tempeh or whole soya beans such as edamame. Also, many of the soya products we consume in the West are from genetically modified soya, so look for 'organic' or 'non-GM' on the packaging.

The 'Clean 15' foods are:

- Asparagus
- Aubergines
- Avocados
- Cabbage
- Cantaloupe
- Cauliflower
- Frozen peas
- Grapefruit
- Kiwi fruits
- Mangoes
- Onions
- Papayas
- Pineapples
- Sweet potatoes
- Sweetcorn

• • •

You will never get as much advice during your life on what you should and shouldn't eat than when you are pregnant. Everyone has an opinion and official advice can change on a regular basis. You can often be made to feel guilty for eating the wrong thing and many women lose confidence in their food choices. Research continues to improve our understanding of food and its effects on the unborn child and although it is important to keep up to date with these developments, it is not good for you or your baby to become too stressed about what you eat.

The main advice given around food safety during pregnancy is to ensure that you do not contract food poisoning or related bacterial diseases. Basic food hygiene and careful cooking should prevent infection and you may find that you follow many of these practices already. Most foods are fine when cooked properly and eaten in moderation.

CHAPTER 7

THE BENEFITS OF SUPPLEMENTS

When it comes to health and nutrition, food comes first, always. Unfortunately, we can no longer rely completely on food alone to provide us with the full nutrient levels we need. As discussed previously in Chapter 1, this is due to a combination of the way that food is produced (think intense farming techniques and lower nutrient levels in the soil), as well as exposure to stress, environmental pollutants and our increasing use of medication (the contraceptive pill and antibiotics, for example). When this shortfall occurs, we can develop subtle nutrient imbalances that can impact on our own health and, when pregnant, that of the unborn baby. Supplements can help to bridge this increasing gap, even when eating a healthy diet, and this is especially true during preconception, pregnancy and breastfeeding.

A NUTRIENT BOOST DURING PREGNANCY

I have found that some women have had marginally sufficient levels of nutrients in order to 'tick over' throughout their life. However, when they fall pregnant, this marginal status is not enough to supply both them and their developing baby. As a result, they can find themselves feeling very tired, experiencing unwanted pregnancy symptoms, such as digestive issues, or fall ill easily with colds and flu. If you follow a vegetarian and vegan diet, you may also find it harder to access all required nutrients during pregnancy. Many women may find it harder to eat as well as they would like in the early part of pregnancy because of morning sickness (see page 104).

Pregnant women are advised to take supplements containing folic acid and, when breastfeeding too, vitamin D, irrespective of their dietary status. Additional supplements, such as iron, may also be necessary if you are found to have low levels in your blood. However, this is the base minimum and many experts, such as myself, would recommend taking a good multivitamin and mineral supplement formulated specifically for pregnancy and breastfeeding, along with an omega-3 supplement. However, you do need to choose supplements wisely.

NOT ALL SUPPLEMENTS ARE THE SAME

Using synthetic 'isolated' forms of nutrients, where the nutrient is provided on its own and not with the 'team-mates' it is naturally found with in food, can throw up a whole host of other concerns. These include toxicity if fat-soluble nutrients such as vitamins A, D, E and K are consumed in high doses, and the 'competitive absorption' between the nutrients. An example of competitive absorption is between calcium and other minerals – high doses of calcium can inhibit the absorption of other minerals such as zinc, magnesium and iron in some cases. These synthetic nutrients come in many different forms. For example, magnesium can be found as magnesium chelate, magnesium glycinate, magnesium citrate and magnesium succinate. However, all these forms have the same integral flaw; they are never found this way in nature and therefore how well our body recognises and metabolises that nutrient in those forms is questionable.

Supplements using nutrients extracted from or grown in food, such as food-state nutrients, do not have this problem. Instead they provide the nutrient in a form as it would be found in real food, thereby enhancing the body's recognition and therefore use of these nutrients. Providing vitamins and minerals in this live, raw and bio-available 'food state' also means that there is lowered toxicity, as you do not need to use high doses to achieve nutritional effectiveness. 'Bio-available' means in a form that your body is able to absorb and use with much greater efficiency. There is no need to take high doses as proffered by synthetic supplement brands, the majority of which, in reality, is excreted by the body.

As a therapist with a keen interest in the biochemistry involved in nutrient absorption, I recommend getting your nutrient sources from food or food-state nutrients whenever possible.

CHECK FOR ADDED INGREDIENTS

Check the ingredients on the labels for added fillers and binders (also called excipients). These are added to products to 'bulk' them out and/or bind them into tablets or capsules. These include 'anti-caking' agents such as magnesium stearate, silicon dioxide, sucrose, acacia gum, microcrystalline cellulose, cornstarch and even talc!

MULTIVITAMINS

A specific supplement for pregnant and breastfeeding women can be a supportive measure if you feel you may not be getting an adequate supply from your diet. Taking them is a good way to get all the key nutrients recommended in this chapter.

B vitamins, especially B12, biotin and choline, are especially important for your unborn baby's brain development. The period from week six of pregnancy to three months after the birth, if you are breastfeeding, appears to be the most sensitive to deficiency. Choline has been shown to protect your unborn baby from developing chronic stress-related illness in later life and should be should be present in pregnancy formulas. Use of a multivitamin and minerals supplement during pregnancy has been shown to reduce general wear and tear of the cells in both the mother and baby, as well as reduce the risk of pre-eclampsia (see page 118) in pregnant women that were classified as overweight or obese (with a body mass index/BMI above 25).

VITAMIN D

The National Institute for Health and Care Excellence (NICE) recommends that all pregnant and breastfeeding women take vitamin D supplements. This is to support healthy skeletal growth in your baby, especially in the last trimester of pregnancy. If your stores are low at this stage, it may impact on your child's bone health in later life. Some studies have shown vitamin D supplementation during pregnancy reduces the risk of allergic symptoms, such as food allergy and atopic dermatitis, as the baby grows into infancy, but these are not conclusive. More recently, optimising levels of vitamin D during pregnancy has been shown to reduce the risk of autoimmune conditions, particularly those that involve the thyroid, such as thyroiditis, as well as childhood atopic diseases, such as eczema.

You are more likely to be deficient in vitamin D if you are overweight, have little exposure to sunlight and if you are of South Asian, African, Caribbean or Middle Eastern descent. If you think you may fall into any of these categories, it is advisable to have your vitamin D levels checked by having a blood test via your GP.

Within the vitamin D family there are four forms: vitamin D1, D2, D3 and D4. Research shows that vitamin D3 is the most active and necessary part of the vitamin D group, but use of D3 is improved if the other forms are present too. You will find all of these to some degree in food sources of vitamin D, such as oily fish (see page 55).

The recommended dose of vitamin D3 is 10 µg and this will often be in your pregnancy multivitamin and minerals supplement if you are taking one. If you are taking a 'food-state' supplement, this will contain all forms of vitamin D, but aim to eat food sources too so that you get a good mix of all four forms of vitamin D.

IRON

A store of around 60 mg of iron is gathered by your baby during the last trimester to be used by the lean tissues in the first six months of life, and recent research suggests that iron stores accrued during this time are influential throughout your child's life. Zinc supports your baby's use of iron in the first six months of pregnancy, so I recommend that you take iron as either part of your pregnancy multinutrient or, if you are taking iron alone, that you take a zinc supplement providing around 5 mg of zinc. Iron deficiency during pregnancy is also thought to influence the risk of the child being autistic because of iron's central role in the early development of the brain and central nervous system.

FOLATE

Folic acid supplement use before and after pregnancy is advisable to reduce the risk of neural tube defects (NTDs), such as spina bifida, caused by a failure of the brain, spine or spinal cord to properly develop in the first few weeks of pregnancy. Ideally you should start taking 400 µg folic acid supplements in the three months prior to conception and until your twelfth week of pregnancy. Folate intake has health benefits beyond these initial 12 weeks too, but the impact it has on NTDs is only in this initial stage.

Folate crosses the placenta better in the natural form found in food such as avocado and dark green leafy vegetables. For this reason, the use of food-sourced folic acid is considered favourable. If you have a history of NTDs from previous pregnancies, or if you are on anti-epileptic medication or if have diabetes, your need for folic acid may be higher and you should discuss this with your medical practitioner or a nutritional therapist. (For further information on the benefits of folates during pregnancy, see page 49.)

OMEGA-3

Fatty acids, DHA especially (see page 41), are vital for the development of normal brain and eye function, especially in the last trimester. There are a number of different types of omega-3 supplements available on the market. Some will provide omega-3 from fish sources, others will provide them from algae or flaxseed (also know as linseed). The latter are suitable for vegans and vegetarians. Omega-3 from fish provides ready-made EPA and DHA that does not need converting before the body can use them. Vegetarian seed sources, such as flaxseed, do need converting, however, and not everyone is able to convert the omega-3 found in the vegetarian forms into the beneficial fatty acids DHA and EPA.

The placenta extracts the DHA and EPA fatty acids from your circulation and then concentrates them in your baby's circulation, so that your baby's levels are twice as high as your own. If you are deficient in these essential fatty acids, your body will begin to extract DHA from its richest store – your brain – so that the baby's supply continues. This may provide an insight into the term 'baby brain', as there is thought to be a 2–3 per cent shrinkage in the mother's brain during pregnancy. This can mean that your concentration is low and you feel forgetful or vague, particularly during the last trimester and while breastfeeding, when the DHA requirement is even higher (it is estimated that the mother passes up to 7 g of fat to her baby through the placenta by the end of the pregnancy). This is where omega-3 supplements providing DHA can become a vital part of your pregnancy scaffolding. They have also been shown to reduce the risk of water retention, dry, itchy skin and stretch marks during pregnancy.

Choose a high-quality fish oil that provides 200–400 mg DHA per daily dose. Omega-3 supplements are screened to ensure they have low level of pollutants. Choose those that are made from smaller fish, such as anchovies and sardines, rather than tuna or salmon – these smaller fish are thought to contain lower level of pollutants. This information should be made clear on the packaging.

BENEFICIAL FLORA

It is now well understood that taking probiotics during pregnancy can increase your baby's immune strength, as well as improve your baby's ability to tolerate lactose once born. Multiple studies show a reduction in infectious and antibiotic-associated diarrhoea from taking Lactobacillus strains, including rhamnosus and casei, both during and after pregnancy if you are breastfeeding. Evidence also suggests that mothers-to-be who take probiotics can reduce the risk of their children developing allergic diseases and conditions such as eczema. At the age of five, there was a 17 per cent decrease in allergenic disease in children whose mothers had taken probiotic supplements in the last trimester and whilst breastfeeding, compared to the placebo group.

Beneficial flora can be of great support to your health too. Some women find that they experience constipation or recurrent thrush during pregnancy, often due to the change in hormone levels, and these conditions can be alleviated by improving the balance of your beneficial flora. A one-month course in addition to your pregnancy multinutrient in the last trimester can be supportive in preparing for birth.

There are a lot of probiotic supplements available. Choose one that offers a mix of different strains (around eight), including Lactobacillus, Bifidobacterium and Streptococcus, as this has been shown to reflect the more natural gut environment. Loose powders that you can add into food or liquids are preferable as they are thought to be used more effectively by the gastro-intestinal system. Some companies also provide probiotics with something called fructooligosaccharides (FOS), a form of prebiotic. Prebiotics 'feed' the beneficial probiotics, but I have found that the addition of these can make some people feel too gassy. If you are eating a diet rich in vegetables, you will be taking in sufficient prebiotics through your diet so may want to choose a product without added prebiotics.

Select a product that contains at least 10 billion colony-forming units (CFU). Probiotics are vulnerable so store your supplements away from bright light and preferably in a cool cupboard or fridge in dark glass jars. If you buy supplements from a high street shop, choose ones that have not have been out under the bright light on a shelf.

HEALTHY START SCHEME

The Healthy Start scheme is an initiative driven by the Department of Health to support pregnant women and women of young children on a low income or under the age of 18. Eligible women are given access to free supplements to support the intake of nutrients, specifically vitamins C, D and folic acid. They are also eligible for vouchers for free fruit, vegetables and milk. Ask your midwife or GP for more information if this applies to you.

TOP TIPS ON FINDING THE RIGHT SUPPLEMENTS

- Choose one that has been specifically formulated for pregnancy.
- Choose one that uses nutrients in as natural a form as possible.
- Choose one that has as little fillers and binders as possible.
- Choose a brand that adheres to the Good Manufacturing Practice (GMP) code of ethics. This will either be detailed on the packaging or you can contact the supplement company directly to ask.

- Don't feel shy about asking the company for more details on the manufacturing process and type of nutrients provided.
- Don't be swayed by cost. Cheap supplements often mean cheap unwanted ingredients.

• • •

There is no substitute for a nutritious, healthy and delicious diet during pregnancy. Food is one of the greatest sensory pleasures, and getting your vitamins and minerals from tasty meals can be a great comfort when you are missing your favourite red wine or exhilarating run.

In an ideal world, your nutritional needs and those of your baby would be met by eating the right macronutrients and micronutrients, but in an age of mass-produced food and busy lifestyles it is not always possible to meet this ideal. Taking supplements is now recommended for all expectant mothers and is no longer seen as an indicator of a poor diet. The quality and efficacy of supplements do vary and so it is important to choose wisely; I always recommend food-state supplements as they are the closest to the natural state found in food.

The science can be overwhelming but by following a balanced diet and by choosing a good multivitamin complex you should be on the right track to a healthy pregnancy for both you and your baby.

CHAPTER 8

EATING WELL WHEN YOU ARE VEGETARIAN OR VEGAN

Different diets have different nutritional strengths and weaknesses, and it is perfectly possible to have a healthy vegetarian diet during pregnancy. Well-balanced vegetarian diets can actually be very beneficial to health and the environment.

During pregnancy, it is important for all women to take a fresh look at their diet, and vegetarians and vegans need to be mindful of some common pitfalls to ensure an adequate consumption of protein, iron, calcium and vitamin B12.

BRIDGING THE GAP

Healthy vegetarian diets tend, by default, to be lower in unhealthy fats and higher in fibre and antioxidants (such as carotenoids, and vitamins C and E) simply because their diets tend to be higher in plant varieties. Because of their relative increase in green leafy vegetables, they also tend to be higher in folate and magnesium (perhaps this is why they have been shown to have a lower incidence of leg cramps in the last trimester). This doesn't, however, alleviate the need for folate supplements (see page 92). The unhealthy vegetarian or vegan diet can also be low in key macronutrient groups, including quality protein and essential fats, as well as micronutrients such as iron, zinc and vitamin B12, all of which are crucial to the healthy development of your unborn baby.

Meat is a source of a number of important nutrients during pregnancy, including protein, the amino acid glycine, iron and vitamin B12. Vegetarians and vegans must therefore source these from other dietary sources. If you are someone who is not strictly vegetarian, but who eats very little red meat, you may also fare well on the advice in this chapter.

By simply being aware of this if you are vegetarian, and by planning your meals carefully, you can have a diet as nutritionally comprehensive as any meat eater.

PROTEIN

Protein requirements increase in pregnancy and breastfeeding and should make up approximately 20 per cent of your daily diet. A varied vegetarian or vegan diet can easily accommodate this because protein is also found in pulses and grains; for non-vegans in eggs and, if you are a pescetarian, in fish.

SOURCES OF 'COMPLETE' PLANT-BASED PROTEINS

- Soya beans and soya products (e.g. tempeh, tofu)
- Quinoa
- Amaranth
- Buckwheat
- Chlorella
- Spirulina

VEGETARIAN SOURCES OF ANIMAL PROTEINS

- Eggs (preferably free-range or organic)
- Dairy products

You can also mix other proteins, called 'protein combining', to create a complete protein. Many cultures that traditionally follow a vegetarian way of eating use this method of 'protein combining'. This can be done by mixing two of any of these three groups:

Whole grains	Nuts/seeds	Legumes
Brown rice	Sunflower, sesame, hemp and pumpkin	Chickpeas
Barley	Seed sprouts	Peas
Rye	Almonds	Black-eyed beans
Millet	Walnuts	Kidney beans
Oats	Cashew nuts	Bean sprouts
Wholegrain pasta	Nut butters (e.g. almond)	

Examples of these combinations include:

- Tofu, Spinach and Walnut Loaf (see page 185) with brown rice
- Chickpea houmus on rye bread
- Nut butter on oatcakes
- Open rye sandwich with houmus and sprouted alfalfa seeds
- Vegetable and black-eyed bean stir-fry with cashew nuts and brown rice noodles

Try to mix all of these rather than relying on one food source such as dairy. Instead include complete and combined plant proteins in your diet.

Ideally, combine these foods within one meal as this increases your body's use of these amino acids by over 30 per cent. However, ensuring you cover two of the three categories within your daily diet will be sufficient.

VITAMIN B12

Although vitamin B12 is primarily derived from animal sources, some sources are suitable for vegetarians too, including eggs, milk, yoghurt, nutritional yeast (such as brewer's yeast), yeast extract and cheese. If you are vegan, you need to consider supplementing with a B12 supplement derived from B12-enriched yeasts, bacterial fermentation or algae. You will also find that some foods such as rice milk and cereals are 'fortified' with vitamin B12, although this is not the ideal source of B12 (see page 52).

IRON

There are two forms of iron: haem and non-haem. Animal products, including eggs, provide the haem form of iron and this is well utilised by your body. Vegetables, including green leafy vegetables such as spinach, however, provide the non-haem form and this is less well absorbed. To compensate for this, vegetables are a rich source of vitamin C and this improves the way your body uses iron. Over-boiling vegetables decreases this iron availability by up to 20 per cent, so cook them mindfully.

Other non-haem sources of iron include brewer's yeast, wheat-germ, wholemeal bread, dried organic fruit (such as prunes and apricots), parsley, cocoa and some curry powders.

Some plant fibre that includes phytates and oxalates (see page 62) can decrease your body's absorption of minerals, including iron, and therefore soaking them or steaming them (in the case of spinach) prior to eating them can increase the iron content. Coffee and the tannins found in tea and raw cacao can also reduce absorption, so don't drink these around mealtimes or when taking iron supplements.

CALCIUM

If you are following a vegan diet and cutting out dairy foods you can run a higher risk of calcium deficiency during pregnancy. A high-fibre vegetarian diet can also increase this risk if you do not soak your pulses and grains appropriately (see page 62). However, it is still possible to obtain calcium from other vegetarian sources – milk, cheese, yoghurt, fromage frais and eggs – and vegan sources, including all nuts, seeds (especially sesame seeds), pulses (soaked or sprouted) and green leafy vegetables. Combining these with sources rich in magnesium and vitamin D will also increase the supply to you and your unborn baby.

Magnesium and vitamin D are essential for the absorption of calcium. However, as discussed in Chapter 5, the plant form of vitamin D – vitamin D2 – is not as efficiently absorbed as the animal sourced D3. Vegetarians can still get their vitamin D from eggs, cow's milk, butter and soy milk. Vitamin D supplements (see page 91) are recommended for all pregnant and breastfeeding women, but are particularly important for those who are vegan.

ZINC

Meat is a rich source of zinc and therefore those who don't eat it can run a higher risk of zinc deficiency. Non-meat sources include brewer's yeast, whole grains, all nuts, seeds (especially pumpkin), dark green leafy vegetables, pulses, eggs and cheese. Zinc absorption can be reduced by the phytates found in pulses so soaking them overnight will help to get the best nutritional benefit.

ESSENTIAL FATTY ACIDS

Vegetarians have been found to have a low intake of omega-3 fats, which, as we know, are very important for you and your baby during pregnancy. Flaxseed and walnuts are excellent sources but not everyone finds it easy to convert these into the important fatty acids DHA and EPA (see page 41). As vegetarians and vegans obtain their omega-3 from plant or seed sources, their breast milk has been shown to be lower in these key fatty acids and this is why the

Vegetarian Society suggests supplementing your diet with a DHA-rich algae supplement provided in a non-gelatin capsule. Another issue is that vegetarians and vegans tend to have a higher intake of omega-6, which we also know can inhibit your body's use of omega-3. To improve this, use coconut oil to cook with rather than sunflower oil.

WAYS TO ACHIEVE A HEALTHY VEGETARIAN PREGNANCY DIET

- Eat a varied diet.
- Eat home-made foods and reduce pre-packaged and processed 'protein alternatives'.
- Eat three portions of whole grains per day (a portion is 1 tablespoon of cooked brown rice or 1 slice of wholemeal bread, for example).
- Steam your green vegetables.
- Eat at least five portions of vegetables of varying colours a day (around 400 g/14 oz).
- Eat around two portions of vitamin C-rich fruit a day, such as berries (approximately 2–3 tablespoons of mixed berries).
- Add organic dried fruit to your breakfast and salads, or eat as a snack.
- Add nuts and seeds to meals – sprinkle on salads, on top of soups, add to stir fries, and eat as a snack. Aim for round 30 g (1 oz) a day.
- Aim for 2–3 servings of pulses per day.
- Use butter on your crackers and bread.
- Drink half a pint of organic non-GM soya milk a day or eat 200 g/7 oz of plain live yoghurt.
- Be aware that textured vegetable protein (TVP) and mycoprotein are acceptable sources of protein occasionally but aim to eat no more than twice a week.

- Use nut and seed butter, which is like a spread, as a snack with apple or chopped pear. Add it into smoothies.
- Add a protein powder, such as hemp, pea or rice, into a smoothie.

MEAT CRAVINGS IN PREGNANCY

Some women crave meat during pregnancy and therefore eat it or fish. These cravings are often a way of your body letting you know that it needs extra iron or B12. If you don't want to eat meat or fish, you could try increasing your intake of vegan or vegetarian sources of these foods such as fermented foods (see the Sauerkraut recipe on page 206) or brewer's yeast for a few weeks to see if the craving subsides.

• • •

Vegetarian or not, the principles remain the same: a healthy diet is composed of non-processed, fresh and varied ingredients complemented where needed by good food-state supplements. By using the information found in this chapter there is no reason why vegans and vegetarians should not have a healthy pregnancy and birth.

CHAPTER 9

MANAGING COMMON PREGNANCY SYMPTOMS

Very few women manage to escape health conditions during pregnancy. Even the healthiest women may suffer from a little bit of nausea, usually within the early weeks. Nausea is often the first tell-tale sign that a woman has conceived, but most go on to have a healthy and radiant pregnancy, especially if they are eating and resting well. Most complaints are not serious, but can cause discomfort, such as constipation, and may make you feel a little down. The good news is that many of these ailments can be easily treated by making dietary changes and by taking nutritional supplements. In this chapter I will discuss the common pregnancy complaints and the small changes to your diet that can make a difference.

MORNING SICKNESS

Morning sickness is not, as the name suggests, limited to the morning. In fact, many women, myself included, experience it at the end of the day, triggered by tiredness or a long period without eating. Pungent smells such as tobacco smoke, fried food or strong perfumes can also trigger queasiness.

Ninety per cent of pregnant women are thought to experience some degree of morning sickness during their pregnancy – 30 per cent of these may experience severe nausea accompanied by vomiting.

General symptoms are unrelenting nausea, sometimes, although not always, accompanied by vomiting and an unpleasant taste in the mouth (some women describe it as a metallic or mouldy taste). It is attributed to the changing levels of a hormone called human chorionic gonadotropin (hCG) in the bloodstream, particularly in the first trimester when the change is at its most rapid, peaking at weeks 9–10 but reducing again at around weeks 12–14. If you are carrying twins, the level of this hormone is even higher and therefore symptoms may be greater. Morning sickness is also exacerbated and contributed to by a drop in blood sugar (see page 24) and deficiencies in zinc and vitamin B6. Up to 40 mg of vitamin B6 (pyridoxine) is considered safe and can be effective at reducing symptoms.

The silver lining is that 'morning' sickness can actually be a good sign; a sign that your hormone levels are changing as they should to ensure a healthy pregnancy. Equally, if you are not experiencing morning sickness, don't worry – you may just be one of the lucky 10 per cent of pregnant women who escape it!

If you are actually vomiting, you need to ensure that you are keeping well hydrated (see tips, page 107) and that you are eating plenty of foods rich in magnesium, as this mineral is lost through vomiting. If you are vomiting frequently throughout the day and unable to hold food or water down, you may be experiencing hyperemesis gravidarum, a condition known to affect 2 per cent of women that ultimately requires hospital treatment to avoid dangerous levels of dehydration. In my experience, this condition is more common in women with gastrointestinal dysfunction, infection with the parasite helicobacter pylori or those who have a thyroid imbalance. Supplementing with 1.5 mg of vitamin B1 per day under medical supervision has also shown to be effective in some cases. However, this does not correct hydration and this must be monitored through your GP or a hospital. Complementary practices such as acupuncture and hypnosis have also been shown to be supportive.

Insufficient levels of digestive enzymes, bile and hydrochloric acid that are needed to break down food, have also been associated with a higher vulnerability to experiencing morning sickness. A qualified nutritional therapist or naturopath will be able to help you determine whether this may be the case by doing a simple test with a solution of water and bicarbonate of soda (see box, page 109). Some signs to look out for are bloating after meals, strong belching after eating, feeling full very quickly (note that this also occurs simply from the size of your baby towards the end of the pregnancy), trouble digesting fatty foods or a history of skin conditions such as eczema and psoriasis.

Ginger root is a traditional remedy for morning sickness because of its action on the gastrointestinal tract, as well on the signalling in the brain that controls vomiting reflexes. In a review published in *Obstetrics & Gynecology*, 1 g per day of fresh ginger root over four days was shown to significantly reduce symptoms for women with mild morning sickness and in women experiencing hyperemesis gravidarum. Ginger is also a source of zinc, and zinc deficiency is associated with morning sickness. During all three of my pregnancies, I have lived on Ginger Chews, available in most health food stores. You can find other brands, but check the packets for added sugars.

Acupuncture and homeopathy have been effective for some of my clients. Commonly used homeopathic remedies are nux vomica 30c, pulsatilla 30c, and ipecac 30c, but remedies are best prescribed by a professional, registered homeopath (see page 217).

WAYS TO HELP YOUR MORNING SICKNESS

- Eat every 2–3 hours to maintain healthy blood-sugar levels.
- Include protein with every meal and snack.
- Eat something dry, such as oatcakes or a rye cracker, as soon as you get up. If you can get your partner to make you a freshly grated ginger in hot water with lemon, this is even better.

- If you cannot tolerate much liquid, you could try sucking home-made fruit lollies or frozen ice cubes of apple juice. Some women also find sucking on a lemon helpful.
- Try a ginger lozenge or chew, such as Ginger Chews.
- Avoid eating fatty, greasy foods as these are harder to digest and can trigger nausea.
- Try drinking a capful of apple cider vinegar in hot water through-out the day.
- Ensure you are drinking plenty of water: 6–8 glasses (including herbal tea or lemon and hot water).
- Minimise your exposure to stress as this has been shown to worsen symptoms.
- Grate fresh ginger into your meals.
- Get fresh air regularly throughout the day. If you are at work, take a break mid-morning and mid-afternoon to go for a quick 10-minute stroll, even if it is raining. This is important for circulation, too.
- You may benefit from taking additional vitamin B6 (see page 105).
- Consider taking some Swedish bitters to improve your digestion of protein, fats and carbohydrates.

HEADACHES AND MIGRAINES

Severe headaches can be common in the first trimester. Again these are thought to be attributed to fluctuating hormone levels. Simply being pregnant can cause tension, which is commonly felt in the muscles, particularly in the neck and shoulders. Normally a painkiller will suffice, but during pregnancy you cannot take painkillers other than paracetamol, particularly in the first trimester, to relieve the tension.

Keeping your blood-sugar levels stable (see page 24) is very important in both the prevention and cure of headaches in pregnancy. Make sure you eat little and often. You can find that you have a greater need for hydration during pregnancy and not catering for this can cause dehydration, which can lead to headaches.

Massage by a qualified masseuse can also help. Alternatively, I found gently massaging my temple and the area from the bridge of my nose across to the ends of my eyebrows with some almond oil helped greatly. Regular yoga practice (see Chapter 13), homeopathy and acupuncture can also be very supportive. Some have also found herbalism and reflexology helpful.

HEARTBURN

This is another classic symptom of pregnancy and tends to be more common in the last trimester. During pregnancy, the muscle valve that usually prevents foods from the stomach going back into the oesophagus becomes more relaxed because of hormonal changes. As your baby grows, the increasing growth can also put extra pressure on this area and exacerbate symptoms. This will ease as your baby's head engages and therefore moves down, which can occur earlier in first pregnancies but much later in subsequent ones.

If you experienced a bit of heartburn before the pregnancy, your symptoms may also be due to imbalances in your stomach acid. GPs and patients alike can sometimes wrongly assume that acidic burning can be a result of too much stomach acid and are therefore prescribed antacids. However, in many cases, the reverse is actually the problem – you are actually secreting too little stomach acid. Antacids only perpetuate the problem in the long run by inhibiting the stomach acid release. This stomach acid is also responsible for the absorption of many minerals, including calcium and zinc, so healthy stomach acid secretion is important in pregnancy. Another contributory factor can be the presence of helicobacter pylori, which a nutritional therapist or your GP can help you to diagnose through a stool test.

WAYS TO EASE YOUR HEARTBURN

- It can be considerably worse after eating larger meals, so reduce your portion sizes.
- Don't drink too much liquid in one go or with meals.
- Sit upright as much as possible, rather than slouching, especially when eating.
- Exercise throughout pregnancy to help support muscle tone.
- Eat plenty of green leafy vegetables – they are rich in magnesium and this mineral is needed for healthy muscle contractions.
- Eat light, simple meals in the morning.
- Sleep in a slightly raised position with pillows softly supporting you.
- Avoid very fatty or spicy foods. Citrus fruits, such as oranges, can also be problematic.
- Add lemon or apple cider vinegar into your food. These actually become alkaline on ingestion, helping to moderate excess acidity if this is the problem.
- Eat live yoghurt as this can be soothing and cooling for the oesophagus.

THE NATUROPATHIC ASSESSMENT OF STOMACH ACID

Mix a quarter of a teaspoon of baking soda or bicarbonate of soda into a small glass of water. Drink the mixture first thing in the morning before eating or drinking anything. If you burp within five minutes, your hydrochloric acid levels are fine; if you do not, they could be too low. A qualified nutritional therapist or naturopath will be able to help you improve this.

CONSTIPATION

Constipation can be another symptom of the muscles relaxing during pregnancy, primarily due to an increase in progesterone levels. The muscles in your gut move food along by a contracting and releasing mechanism called peristaltic movement. If this function relaxes, food is not passed as effectively through the digestive tract and into the rectum to be eliminated. Towards the last trimester, the weight of the baby on your bowels can make this even more intense.

Prescription iron tablets often use ferrous sulphate as the form of iron and this can cause constipation and black stools. Encouraging a daily bowel movement is very important as, similar to a dustbin, if you leave food in there for too long it can start to cause other problems, including reducing absorption of nutrients from your food. Progesterone suppositories can also cause constipation, uncomfortable wind and bloating. Too much pressure can also result in haemorrhoids (see page 111).

Constipation can also be related to your emotional health. The gut is also referred to as 'the second brain', a term coined by Dr Michael Gershon, a neuro-gastroenterologist. This is because the gut has over 100 million neurons and houses the largest collection of neural tissue in the body (after the brain) called the enteric nervous system (ENS). This inextricable link between the brain and the gut means that emotions such as anxiety, fear and excitement are also felt in your gut, hence the term 'butterflies in your stomach' or 'gut instinct'. The point of this is that your emotional health may also be affecting the function of your gut and therefore can be associated with 'holding on' and constipation.

WAYS TO EASE CONSTIPATION

- Try soaking a tablespoon of flaxseed in half a tumbler of water. Leave for half an hour and then drink the liquid and mixture in one go (it can be quite gloopy). Try drinking the mixture at night when you are more relaxed – it usually encourages a trip to the loo in the morning.

- Eat plenty of vegetables as these are rich in fibre as well as water.
- Drink plenty of water and herbal teas, at least 6–8 glasses a day. You will probably find that your thirst increases through pregnancy and breastfeeding as your water requirement increases.
- Do regular, gentle exercise such as yoga (see Chapter 13), swimming and walking to help strengthen peristaltic movement.
- Consider switching your iron tablets to a gentler more natural version, which do not tend to cause constipation.
- Avoid eating processed or sugary foods as these can cause the stagnant faecal matter to ferment and cause further problems.
- Chop prunes or add prune juice to your breakfast.
- Consider having homeopathy, acupuncture and massage.
- Consider ways to reduce your stress, such as gentle exercise and more 'quiet time' without technology if you feel this might be influencing your bowel movements.

HAEMORRHOIDS AND VARICOSE VEINS

Haemorrhoids – or piles – can be caused by constipation. During pregnancy the veins are under more pressure to circulate the increasing blood volume. The blood can collect in the veins causing them to swell and protrude, commonly in the rectum, vulva or lower legs. The pressure on trying to pass a bowel movement in combination with the increasing weight of your baby can cause the veins to swell, causing haemorrhoids. This can cause itching and pain on attempting a bowel movement. It can also cause a small amount of bleeding, but if this becomes a lot of blood or more frequent, seek medical advice. Similarly, varicose veins can occur from the increase in overall weight and blood volume, which can cause the blood vessels in your legs to enlarge.

WAYS TO PREVENT AND HELP HAEMORRHOIDS AND VARICOSE VEINS

- Eat foods rich in vitamin C, such as plenty of fruit and vegetables.
- Eat foods rich in compounds called anthocyanidins, which are found in all berries.
- Tackle any constipation using the tips on page 110.
- Rest regularly, placing your legs at a 90-degree angle.
- Do gentle exercise such as yoga (see Chapter 13), swimming or walking to support healthy circulation.
- Bath in Epsom salts – pour the salts into a warm bath and rest there for 20 minutes.

STRETCH MARKS

The skin around your middle has to do a great job of stretching as your baby grows. Sometimes this expansion goes beyond the abilities of your skin's elastin (this is what makes your skin 'elastic' or stretchy). When this happens, you can develop stretch marks. These are most commonly found around the stomach, hips, thighs and breasts. Moisturising daily may help, but your skin is often an illustration of what is going on inside your body and stretch marks can also be a sign of zinc, vitamin C, vitamin E or omega-3 fatty acid deficiency. Vitamins C and E help your body to make the elastin that is needed for growth, and omega-3 fats help to keep the skin moisturised from the inside out.

WAYS TO MINIMISE STRETCH MARKS

- Eat foods rich in vitamins E and C, such as berries, avocados and green leafy vegetables.
- Build zinc-rich foods, such as pumpkin seeds, lamb and natural yoghurt, into your diet as often as you can.
- Take an omega-3 supplement to support your intake of essential fatty acids.

● Moisturise your skin daily with vitamin E-rich oil, such as avocado oil. This is especially helpful in the last weeks of pregnancy and after birth to encourage the skin to contract.

RESTLESS LEGS OR LEG CRAMPS

This can be common in the last trimester and can be worse at night, causing insomnia and the inability to sit still or rest. The cause of restless leg syndrome (RLS) isn't known, but it has been associated with low dopamine levels, a brain chemical that has a lot of important functions in the body. As iron is needed for the production of dopamine, low iron has also been associated with RLS, and deficiency appears to be more common in pregnancy for women who have low iron levels. Symptoms reduce when iron levels are improved. Low folic acid levels have also been associated with RLS but the link is less known. Leg cramps can be a sign of not having enough magnesium, calcium or potassium, which can create spasms in the leg.

WAYS TO EASE RLS

● Increase your intake of green leafy vegetables as these are rich in iron, magnesium and folic acid, as well as sesame seeds, sardines and apricots.
● Add some light dairy foods, such as yoghurt, to your diet to increase your calcium and magnesium intake.
● You may benefit from taking additional iron supplements (see page 92).
● Bath in Epsom salts as this provides magnesium.

INSOMNIA

Sleep can be affected at different stages of pregnancy for different reasons. Towards the end of your pregnancy you may find that you are woken up regularly to go to the loo or because of movement from your growing baby. In the early stages it may be due to the hormonal changes that are occurring, as well as possible anxiety about this next step in your life. It is my belief that sleep becomes lighter towards the end of your pregnancy in preparation for birth and to prepare you for waking in the night to feed your new baby.

You may also be experiencing a degree of anticipation around labour and new parenthood towards the end of your pregnancy. In some traditional practices it is believed that the womb is connected to the heart and that pregnancy can increase anxiety, which can also affect sleep. Be gentle on yourself and allow yourself to express these perfectly natural emotions. Ask for comfort from those around you and talk to your partner about your concerns.

WAYS TO GET A BETTER NIGHT'S SLEEP

- Bath in Epsom salts before bed. These provide magnesium, a deficiency of which can contribute to insomnia.
- Try sprinkling lavender essential oil drops on your pillow.
- Don't eat late at night as going to sleep on a full stomach can cause you to sleep lightly. This can also cause heartburn. Try to eat a minimum of 2½ hours before going to bed.

OEDEMA

This is the swelling of the ankles and hands caused by retained fluid. It can be contributed to by hormonal changes, mineral deficiencies and a diet that is high in sugar or salty foods. Don't be tempted to reduce your water intake. Ironically, dehydration can also cause water retention, so increasing your fluids can actually reduce oedema.

WAYS TO EASE OEDEMA

- Eat asparagus, artichokes, celery, parsley, cabbage and black-currants, as these are natural diuretics.

- Choose rock or sea salt rather than table salt.
- Drink dandelion leaf or nettle tea as they are natural diuretic teas.
- Avoid eating food that is high in salt and sugar.

CARPAL TUNNEL SYNDROME

This condition, common in pregnancy, affects the nerves in the wrist and can result in tingling or numbness in the fingers. It may get worse at night. Carpal tunnel syndrome has been associated with low levels of B vitamins, particularly vitamin B12. Your midwife will refer you to a GP for advice if you experience this condition, or you can read more about how to deal with it through exercises on the NHS website (see page 213).

It is advisable to increase your intake of B vitamin foods such as bananas, chickpeas, egg yolks, wholemeal bread, sesame seeds and yeast extract.

THRUSH

Some women can be vulnerable to thrush during pregnancy, which is in part due to the change in oestrogen that makes the vagina rich in a type of sugar called glycogen. This glycogen feeds a natural yeast that is present in the vagina and gut called Candida albicans, which then 'overgrows' and causes the symptoms of thrush such as itchiness, soreness or redness around the vagina, It may produce a thick, white or creamy texture that smells of yeast. However, a diet that is low in fibre and high in sugary foods also feeds the growth of candida albicans. A healthy level of beneficial flora (see page 94) can usually keep this in check, but if you had a diet that was high in these foods, such as sweets, chocolate and white bread, or you had an imbalance in beneficial flora before you fell pregnant, you can be more likely to experience thrush during pregnancy.

It is especially important to address this prior to giving birth as during the natural birth process, your baby will ingest the flora that is present in your vaginal canal. This is the amazing process designed by nature that builds the baby's immune system. However, this can also mean that they are also likely to ingest the overgrowth of Candida albicans if it is present and this can increase the incidence of thrush in your baby, for example. Candida albicans is also an iron-loving yeast and may make you more susceptible to iron-deficiency anaemia in pregnancy.

WAYS TO EASE THRUSH

- Put a couple of teaspoons of natural live yoghurt on a sanitary towel in your underwear.
- Avoid using perfumed soaps. Natural glycerine-based soaps are less irritating and, with the inclusion of ingredients such as natural aloe vera or calendula, can actually be very healing.
- Add half a cup of apple cider vinegar into a small amount of warm bath water and soak for 10 minutes.
- Support your gut flora with a probiotic supplement. The strain Saccharomyces boulardii has been shown to be particularly effective at reducing overgrowth of Candida albicans and is safe to take during pregnancy. It has also been shown to be as effective as the prescription anti-fungal drug Nystatin at reducing the incidence of Candida albicans overgrowth in babies, especially those that are pre-term.
- Increase your intake of fibre from vegetables, especially those rich in prebiotics such as artichokes, asparagus, chicory, garlic and onions.
- Avoid eating foods containing refined sugar or refined carbohydrates.
- Consult a qualified nutritional therapist or naturopath to help you address the reasons why overgrowth may have occurred in the first place (see page 216).

- Eat plenty of iron-rich foods, such as blackstrap molasses and green leafy vegetables.

GESTATIONAL DIABETES

Gestational diabetes is high blood sugar developed during pregnancy that subsides after pregnancy. It is thought to affect around 5 per cent of pregnant women and is not life-threatening, but it can lead to a higher risk of high blood pressure. It is usually detected in the second trimester, at around 24 weeks.

The condition means that your baby will receive more glucose, and therefore more calories and be 'big for gestational age', which can lead to a Caesarean birth. However, there is much that can be done to control gestational diabetes and therefore reduce your baby's risk of developing problems with weight and blood-sugar handling in later life too. At the time of writing, new research suggests that the time at which gestational diabetes presents itself is key in determining the impact the condition will have on the baby's health. If it is developed and controlled in the first trimester, there is a lower chance of the baby being big for gestational age at birth but there is still a higher risk of the baby being overweight than in a normal pregnancy.

There is a higher risk of developing gestational diabetes if you have a family history of diabetes, have had large babies before, have a body mass index (BMI) over 30 or if your family history is Middle Eastern, black Caribbean or South Asian. The best protection against gestational diabetes is to follow the guidelines in this book that support healthy blood-sugar management. Robust evidence has shown that a diet rich in fruits, vegetables, whole grains and low-fat dairy products, and low in saturated fats, total fats, cholesterol, refined grains, sweets, and sodium (also known as Dietary Approaches to Stop Hypertension or DASH diet) significantly improves the chance of a healthy pregnancy and baby.

Vitamin D is used for insulin production and an increasing body of research is showing that improving vitamin D intake through supplementation can significantly improve the chances of a healthy pregnancy and baby in women with gestational diabetes. Your midwife will also provide information if you are at risk of or develop gestational diabetes.

You need to be especially vigilant about following the healthy dietary principles outlined in this book. In addition to these, there are lifestyle and dietary strategies that can help:

- The spice cinnamon (preferably use fresh – I use a brand called Cinnamon Hill) has been shown to support glucose metabolism. Add this to food, such as your breakfast, stews, curries and yoghurt.
- The minerals chromium, magnesium, zinc and vitamins B, C, D and K play an important role in glucose management, so look for these to be included in your pregnancy multinutrient. You may also need to take additional vitamin D – a blood test can determine if this is the case.

PRE-ECLAMPSIA

This is a serious pregnancy disorder experienced by around 10 per cent of pregnant women. Symptoms are high blood pressure and protein in the urine. You may also experience blurred vision, swelling and headaches.

You are at a greater risk of developing pre-eclampsia if you are carrying more than one baby, are over 35 years of age, overweight or have a family history of the condition. It is related to problems in the development of the placenta. Treated early, it can cause no harm but if left untreated it can impact on your health and that of your baby quite seriously. It is the reason why your blood pressure is monitored regularly throughout pregnancy.

There has been some preliminary research into whether or not higher levels of inflammation in the body during pregnancy may be contributing to the development of pre-eclampsia. If this is the case, the dietary principles that you will be following in this book promote foods rich in natural anti-inflammatory properties.

It also appears that women with pre-eclampsia have lower levels of magnesium in their blood. This has led to research showing that increasing magnesium intake through diet and supplements can prevent the onset, and reduce inflammation and symptoms, of pre-eclampsia. Taking pregnancy multivitamins has been shown to help reduce the risk of pre-eclampsia. Similarly, supplementing with Co-enzyme Q10 has also been seen to reduce the risk of developing pre-eclampsia in women at risk of the condition.

WAYS TO REDUCE YOUR RISK OF PRE-ECLAMPSIA

- Avoid having table salt and be mindful of having too much rock or sea salt.
- Increase your intake of potassium-rich and magnesium-rich foods, such as dark green leafy vegetables, squash, fish, yoghurt, avocados and ripe bananas.
- Consult a qualified nutritionist or naturopath to discuss your supplement needs.
- Rest as much as possible.

• • •

Some common pregnancy ailments are a handy sign of vitamin deficiencies and are easily solved with a small dietary changes and by taking food-state supplements. The infuriating symptoms of restless leg syndrome, for example, may highlight an iron deficiency vital for the cognitive development of your child and the production of healthy red blood cells. Not all conditions or complaints can be totally alleviated, but in the case of morning sickness and diabetes, these can sometimes be controlled by changes to the diet; in other cases, medical support may be needed. Where many prescription drugs and treatments are not allowed during pregnancy, complementary therapies such as acupuncture or homeopathy can also offer support for the common complaints during pregnancy (see page 217 for more details).

Every pregnancy is different but by maintaining a nutritious diet and listening to your body, you can help to make your pregnancy as comfortable and as healthy as possible.

CHAPTER 10

NUTRITION TO PREPARE YOU FOR LABOUR

Although your baby's growth ebbs and flows during the first six months of pregnancy, your nutrient requirements remain pretty stable. However, in the final trimester, and in particular in the weeks before the birth, building up a greater nutritional store can be a huge support to you and your baby. This chapter will guide you through this period, as you head towards the end of your pregnancy journey, and help you to prepare your body for birth and support your nutritional needs during labour.

PREPARING FOR BIRTH

The precious weeks before birth are a vulnerable time, characterised by a heady mix of excitement and anticipation, bringing us the closest we may have come before to our deepest emotions. During the last trimester you may find that your energy lessens, and emotional ups and downs intensify. This is completely normal and, where you can, allow it to happen – rest when you feel like it, and cry and laugh when you feel like it too. You may also begin to experience the well-known 'nesting' instinct, which is the desire to get everything in order, tie up loose ends and essentially prepare for the birth. I have even known clients to house-hunt in these weeks, with a sense of urgency to move house once the baby is born! These instincts are all natural, but do remember to slow down too. It is a natural time of nurture and conservation, to build up vital energy stores for labour and the healing process post birth and the all-important production of breast milk.

ESSENTIAL NUTRITION

You might be tempted to think that diet doesn't matter in these final stages, that you've been 'good' for so long, but remember this is about building a way of eating that you can carry on beyond pregnancy that will support you not just physically, but mentally and emotionally too.

Build in time to allow your body to rest and restore at the end of each day. There is a real surge of growth again during the last trimester of pregnancy and this rapid development requires around 400 more calories each day than the usual non-pregnant calorie requirement. This is best achieved by eating little and often, rather than having three big meals. The extra room your baby is taking up and the fact that your digestion can slow down in pregnancy makes big meals harder to digest. These extra calories are a way of building up energy and endurance reserves for labour.

Although labour is a unique experience for each woman, it is, as the word suggests, hard work for most of us and, like every endurance exercise, requires training and preparation – physically and mentally. (See Chapter 13 for ways to support your mind during this final part of the pregnancy journey.)

Your intake of protein and omega-3 fatty acids is particularly important during this trimester. Your protein requirement increases to around 50 g/2 oz per day (see box, page 123). Glycine, an amino acid found in protein, is essential for growth, the immune system and for building energy stores in these last few weeks.

Both your need and your baby's need for zinc mildly increases in the last trimester to around 20 mg per day. Build in zinc-rich foods, including green leafy vegetables, pumpkin seeds, sesame seeds, lentils, almonds, whole grains and lamb.

WHERE TO FIND YOUR EXTRA PROTEIN SOURCES

- 100 g/3½ oz chicken and fish (21–28 g/¾–1 oz)
- 2 eggs (14 g/½ oz)
- 300 ml (½ pint) milk (10 g)
- 200 g/7 oz baked beans (11 g)
- 100 g/3½ oz chickpeas/kidney beans (7 g)
- 1 tablespoon nut or seed butter (3 g)
- 1 small pot of yoghurt (7g)

Ensuring you have adequate iron stores is important too, and this will be checked by your midwife. Do let her know if you are feeling particularly tired, run-down or are losing hair, as these can be signs of iron-deficiency anaemia. See page 59 for how to include more iron-rich foods into your diet.

From 36 weeks, you can start to drink raspberry leaf tea, traditionally used to support the tone of the uterine muscles and ripen the cervix in preparation for birth. Raspberry leaf tea is rich in vitamin C, which is needed for adequate healing and to support the immune system to fight off infection.

NATURAL SUPPORT FOR YOUR BIRTH HORMONES

The production of birth hormones, such as beta-endorphin, oxytocin and prolactin, which stimulate the stages of labour and breastfeeding are dependent on the vitamins and minerals found in your diet. These hormones require vitamin C in the last month of pregnancy – good sources are citrus fruits, kiwi fruits, green leafy vegetables and squash. The hormones also require copper, zinc and calcium, found in green leafy vegetables, bone broths, dairy products, lamb and beef, as well as B vitamins, especially vitamin

B3, folate, vitamin B6 and vitamin B12. The minerals iron and magnesium found in red meat, green leafy vegetables, lentils and nuts, are active components of the body's production of natural hormones called endorphins. These hormones are our body's own pain-management team and will be released in higher amounts during labour. How well your cells respond to prolactin, oxytocin and endorphins is dependent on sulphur-containing amino acids, and these are found in egg yolks, meat, organ meat and broths (see Chicken Stock or Broth recipe on page 207).

VITAMIN K

Building up your vitamin K stores prior to giving birth is important. This fat-soluble nutrient, although needed in small amounts, is essential for effective blood-clotting. You can find vitamin K in avocados, broccoli, beans, cabbage, lettuce, cauliflower, spinach, watercress and nettle tea.

YOUR STATE OF MIND

How you feel when you approach labour and birth can have a profound impact on the way it progresses and may make an intense labour easier to manage. Stress affects the number and diversity of beneficial bacteria in the digestive tract, and increases the demand for B vitamins, magnesium and vitamin C, for example – these are all important nutrients to support the birth process and healing after the birth. Stress also causes the body to produce adrenaline, which can inhibit the birth process. This is a very primal function to protect the baby from being born into a 'dangerous' environment in the days of caves and sabre-toothed tigers!

Resting as much as possible and really drawing on the support around you can build your psychological scaffolding at this exciting and sometimes daunting transition to parenthood. Don't be afraid to ask for help with chores and cooking. Good rest, good nutrition, and extra help from family and friends is invaluable during this time. The yoga sequence in Chapter 13 may help you to achieve a grounded state of mind in these last few weeks.

FOOD DURING LABOUR

If you have been eating according to the principles in this book, you will have been building up a good reserve of something called glycogen. This is stored in the liver and muscles, and provides vital energy during intense activity, such as labour. During labour, this stored glycogen will provide your uterine muscle cells with the power it will need. This intense activity will also draw on your store of B vitamins, calcium, magnesium, chromium, zinc and Co-enzyme Q10.

The labour process can often initiate a 'clearing' from the digestive tract. For some women this may result in being sick or having diarrhoea, which is a natural preparation for the birth process. This can dehydrate the body quite quickly and so sipping small amounts of water to replenish water stores is important. You can also mix apple or orange juice with water to be sipped during labour, as this provides an easy energy source as well as keeping you hydrated.

Eat light snacks to support glucose levels necessary for energizing you during labour. Good snacks are:

- Fennel and Flaxseed Oatcakes (see page 200) with Creamy Spinach Dip (see page 203)
- Banana
- Small pot of yoghurt
- Handful of dried fruit
- Grapes
- Nourish Bar (see page 210)

Note: If you are given opioid drugs during labour, you will be told not to eat.

THE IMPORTANCE OF BENEFICIAL BACTERIA

In humans, 70 per cent of our immune system resides in the gut tissue. Much of this is made up of beneficial flora, or probiotics. In fact, there are 10 times the amount of bacteria than there are cells in our body, and they have a very powerful influence on our health.

Until recently, it was commonly believed that healthy bacteria was not present within the womb and therefore your baby would not be exposed to this until the birth. It was believed that a baby ingested the healthy bacteria for her immune system when she travelled through the birth canal during labour. However, current research is now questioning this and suggests that healthy bacteria is present in both the placenta and the amniotic fluid during pregnancy. This is directly influenced by the healthy bacteria that is present in your system. This would suggest that your baby's immunity is being developed in the womb, too, and underlines the importance of a healthy diet and of you having healthy levels of beneficial bacteria. This development is thought to occur in the last trimester, as babies born prematurely have lower levels and different varieties of these beneficial bacteria species.

The beginnings of this immune development are then built on during the birth process with the ingestion of beneficial bacteria in the birth canal, and will continue to develop and populate over the next 20 days of your baby's life. If you have a balanced bacterial environment, your baby will be ingesting more beneficial bacteria than non-beneficial, which is obviously ideal. However if this is out of balance, in the case of Candida overgrowth (see page 115), your baby can ingest more non-beneficial than beneficial. Low beneficial flora or raised unwanted bacteria, such as E. coli, as a result of antibiotic use during pregnancy, poor diet or medication use, have been associated with low amounts of some of the important bacterial strains. Taking a probiotic in the last month of your pregnancy can help to rebalance this (see page 94).

Babies born by Caesarean section do not get the opportunity to acquire this beneficial bacteria and studies have shown that they have a very different bacterial variation than those born vaginally. Sally Fallon Morell, author of *The Nourishing Traditions Book of Baby & Child Care*, suggests that all babies born by Caesarean section should receive a supplement of bifidus bacteria even if they are breastfed.

In traditional cultures, in the final weeks of pregnancy, the community supports the mother's preparation for birth by making fermented foods rich in good bacteria, such as kefir, to prepare the birth canal. In the Recipes section I have listed a recipe for sauerkraut (see page 208) and kefir (see page 208), which you may want to have a go at making in advance of the birth of your baby.

YOUR POSTNATAL STORE CUPBOARD

Cooking can be a wonderful way to unwind and slow down in the final weeks of your pregnancy. You can use this time to build your postnatal store cupboard and start making some of the recipes in Chapter 14 to keep in the freezer, so you have a nutritious meal to hand at all times. To prepare your postnatal store cupboard, stock up on:

- Grains, such as brown rice, quinoa and barley
- Porridge oats
- Live yoghurt
- Local or manuka honey
- Ginger
- Bay leaves

- Redbush tea bags
- Turmeric
- Oatcakes or rice cakes
- Fennel seeds or fennel tea bags
- Tins of pulses, such as chickpeas, lentils and cannellini beans
- Organic dried apricots
- Mixed seeds, such as pumpkin, sunflower and sesame
- Sweet potatoes
- Cinnamon
- Fresh chicken stock, to keep in the freezer
- Frozen spinach
- Good-quality butter or coconut butter
- Good-quality olive oil
- Eggs
- Nut butters (I recommend the ones by Meridian or Biona)
- Bags of frozen berries
- Miso sachets for instant soups (I like Clearspring brown or white miso)
- Stewed apples or pears, to keep in the freezer
- Bananas

• • •

Getting ready for labour and the birth of your new baby can be both exciting and daunting. You can use these last few weeks as an opportunity to prepare yourself practically, mentally, physically and emotionally for when the time is right for your labour to begin and the precious days with your baby that follow.

CHAPTER 11

FOODS FOR YOUR RECOVERY FROM BIRTH

Pregnancy is a time to look after yourself, focus on your needs through optimum nutrition and rest, and take life a little more gently. This need does not change once your baby is born – and the three months after the birth are known as the fourth trimester for this very reason.

If you are breastfeeding, a healthy diet is needed to support your milk supply and growing baby. If you choose not to breastfeed, or if it hasn't been possible, then diet is still just as important to support recovery from birth and sleep disruption. A good diet helps the restoration of hormonal balance after pregnancy and replenishes nutrient stores that have been diminished.

RECOVERING FROM BIRTH

Traditional cultures would nourish and feed the new mother for a minimum of the first two weeks after the birth. They would do this by cooking and nurturing the mother and baby, feeding them nutritious foods, such as bone broths, and foods high in fat-soluble nutrients such as vitamin A and E (good examples are avocado and sweet potato) needed for healing. The proteins, electrolytes and collagen found in bone broths support repair and healing, and also provide a source of nutrients, such as choline, to support the production of breast milk.

Other foods that can help to rebuild strength after birth are those that are rich sources of minerals, such as iron and calcium – good sources are green leafy vegetables, oats, millet and pulses. Spices, such as ginger and turmeric, support the immune system after birth and reduce inflammation from the birthing process and healing of scar tissue. Almonds and sesame seeds are high in minerals and are a well-digested form of protein.

Many women find that there is a change to their bowel habits after birth and may experience constipation. The foods mentioned above provide fibre to help prevent this. Following the advice for constipation on page 110 will also help.

IRON

In the last trimester your baby accumulates most of the iron that's needed, drawing on your iron stores in preparation for the oxygenated world he will be born into. If you have been following the principles in this book and supporting your diet with a good-quality pregnancy supplement, you will find your iron levels remain good (unless you were iron-deficient prior to pregnancy but unaware of this). However, the birth process can cause a loss of blood and a need to replenish your stores. Be mindful of eating plenty of iron-rich foods (see page 59) daily, such as wilted spinach, red meat and lentils, as well as good sources of vitamin C, which increases the absorption of iron and wound-healing after the birth.

Your body's ability to use iron is also influenced by your levels of healthy bacteria (see page 126), so eating foods that support this or taking a month's course of probiotics can help. This requirement increases if you had any medication or medical intervention during the birthing process, such as an epidural, antibiotics, anti-inflammatory medication or an anaesthetic.

VITAMIN E

Vitamin E has been shown to support wound healing and is also used to promote hormonal balance. In these early weeks you will experience considerable hormonal changes and eating vitamin E-rich foods can help you regain balance. Foods rich in vitamin E include sunflower seeds, wheatgerm and avocado. You can also apply vitamin E oil to closed wounds to help reduce scarring. Rose oil has similar properties and is a wonderful oil for healing and emotional support – you can add this to a bath or burn it in an aromatherapy oil burner.

ZINC

Zinc is needed for the immune system and healing after birth. It supports the production and therefore the moderation of hormones, which will be very changeable over the next few weeks. It can also have an effect on symptoms of postnatal depression (see page 132). Build plenty of zinc-rich foods, such as nuts, lamb and whole grains, into your diet.

WATER

Drinking plenty of fluids is important. If you are not breastfeeding, you will need to drink around six glasses of water a day, although this can also be in the form of herbal teas (caffeinated tea and coffee doesn't count as these are diuretics). If you are breastfeeding, you will need more than this – be led by your thirst levels. It is common to get a bit 'sweaty' after childbirth for the first six weeks or so, particularly at night. This is perfectly natural as it's the body's way of restoring balance again, but do make sure you are replenishing any lost magnesium or water by keeping up your fluids and intake of green leafy vegetables and seeds.

EATING WELL

Following the dietary principles in this book will support your energy during this time and your immune system's ability to repair well. Eating slowly and well can be tricky, so eat while your baby is asleep, regardless of whether or not they are conventional mealtimes. Eating well is more important than having a tidy house.

Keep it simple – it is at this stage you will reap of the benefits of your postnatal store cupboard (see page 127) and any pre-made frozen dishes. If you give birth during the wintery, damper months, avoid eating lots of cold foods and treat yourself to warming stews and soups. Warming, slow-cooked foods can be very nourishing for the gut and immune system, as well as providing a little bit of comfort. Eating in this way has also been shown to be supportive for postnatal mood too. When blood-sugar levels are unstable and low, depression and anxiety can feel worse.

POSTNATAL DEPRESSION

Postnatal depression is different from the 'baby blues'. The baby blues tend to set in around days 3–5 when your breast milk comes in. You might feel weepy or more sensitive to those around you, as well as anxious and overwhelmed. The baby blues are experienced by many new mothers, but usually pass within a few days at the most.

Postnatal depression, however, is more debilitating and all-consuming. It can leave you feeling lethargic and hopeless, and disinterested in the baby and in taking care of yourself. It can affect appetite and sleep patterns and cause you to cry a lot. It lasts for a number of weeks and can occur at any stage in the first year of motherhood.

Like many women who have postnatal depression, you may feel ashamed or guilty about the way you feel, but it is important to remember that you are not alone and that help is available (see page 213). Around 15 per cent of new mothers experience postnatal depression and the causes can range from sudden changes in hormones to a traumatic birth; or even triggered by previous psychological trauma from your own childhood.

There may also be nutritional factors at play – iron deficiency and low vitamin D levels have been shown to be contributory factors to postnatal depression, and these should be checked by your GP.

OMEGA-3 FATS AND POSTNATAL DEPRESSION

There is a significant body of research underlining the influence that healthy DHA and EPA intake can have on the reduction of symptoms of depression, both on their own and in combination with antidepressant medication. Studies are not conclusive, but there is sufficient evidence to advise that they may help. In one study a 1 per cent increase in the blood levels of DHA related to a 59 per cent decrease in the risk of depressive symptoms postnatally. Studies also show that in countries where fish intake is low, postnatal depression is higher. As unborn babies accumulate an average of 67 mg of DHA per day in the last trimester, this can sometimes be at the cost of our fatty acid stores postnatally. Therefore keeping up your intake of omega-3 fatty acids, DHA and EPA, in the latter stage of pregnancy and in this postnatal period is important.

Studies have shown that supplementing the diet with omega-3 fish oil supplements from the 20th week of pregnancy to three months after the birth, was shown to be beneficial in improving mood. However, these benefits were not seen in those women consuming omega-3 from plants or seeds sources. Therefore if you are vegetarian or vegan, I recommend you support your diet with omega-3 supplements made from algae (see page 93).

Remember that depression is a medical condition and not a sign of poor parenting or weakness. Do ask for help – there will be people who want to listen and support you to find balance again so that you can enjoy your baby and motherhood.

SHOULD I TRY CRANIAL OSTEOPATHY?

Although many people have visited an osteopath at some point in their lives, not many have encountered cranial osteopathy. This is a shame because it is an extremely gentle and effective therapy for the relief of pregnancy and post-birth pressure for both you and your baby. Practitioners are trained to feel the rhythmical shape change that is present in all body tissues, known as the cranial rhythm. Cranial osteopathy helps to identify and release the stresses and tensions throughout the body and head that upset this rhythm.

During pregnancy our bodies undergo an immense strain due to the extra weight we are carrying. This can affect our posture and can cause backache, neck pain and sometimes even sciatica. Softening of the ligaments due to hormones can further increase your susceptibility to undue pressure. Not only does cranial osteopathy help to alleviate these tensions, it can also be used to help ensure that the mother's pelvis is structurally balanced by releasing old injuries. If the pelvis is in good shape, the likelihood of an uncomplicated birth and a quick recovery is improved.

We often talk of the impact of childbirth on the mother's body but the baby undergoes a level of trauma too. Birth can be one of the most stressful events of our lives. The baby's head is subject to a lot of force during birth and often emerges misshapen. This corrects itself within a few days, but if this process is not complete the baby may experience discomfort and sleepless nights. Treating the compression in the head during their infancy can diminish the impact of these stresses during later life. Cranial osteopathy is also used on babies who have trouble feeding or are suffering with colic. See the Resources section, page 219 for more information.

WEIGHT LOSS

If you have gained excess weight during pregnancy, don't rush to lose it or reduce your calorie intake. This will only leave you feeling tired and rob you and your baby of precious nutrients, as well as affect your ability to produce breast milk. It is also counterproductive to weight loss and can encourage greater fat storage in the long term.

Even when you are eating the additional 500 calories per day needed during breastfeeding (see page 138), you are still likely to lose around 450–900 g (1–2 lb) a week until you reach your natural weight. This is because looking after a baby and breastfeeding burns a lot of energy!

I encourage you to put the focus on eating wholesome, unrefined real food, using it as a source of whole-body nourishment and strength-building for you and your baby in the first three months, rather than being too concerned with calories.

EXERCISE

Regular exercise after you have been given the all-clear at your six-week check, in combination with the dietary principles in this book, will help you find a healthy weight naturally. However, if you are breastfeeding avoid strenuous exercise for the first 3–6 months. Breastfeeding women who do regular strenuous exercise have been shown to be low in vitamin B6, an important vitamin for restoring hormonal balance as well as supporting serotonin production and energy. Instead opt for gentler practices such as yoga (see Chapter 13) or Pilates, which can be done in class or in the comfort of your own home. The Department of Health recommends doing 30 minutes a day of some form of exercise for five days a week. I found walking a great way to achieve this, as well as supporting my mental and emotional well being.

• • •

There is a lot of pressure in the West for new mothers to get back on their feet and back to normal as quickly as possible, to be seen to be coping well having regained their pre-pregnancy figure. Be kind to yourself and don't be too self-critical. Your body has been through an incredible workout and you deserve a rest. This may be difficult at times, especially if you have other children, but don't be afraid to ask your numerous visitors to lend a hand when needed. Although you have a new and exciting member of the family who is your priority, your health and well-being are of paramount importance too. As a relaxed and well-nourished mother, you will find it much easier to care for your new baby and fully enjoy these precious, early months of your child's life.

CHAPTER 12

FOODS TO BOOST
BREASTFEEDING

There has been a significant increase in the rates of breastfeeding over recent years, which is great news for our babies' health. Due to recent controversies over mothers nursing in public, however, the subject can be very emotive and discussion about it can be polarised and sometimes acrimonious. Many women feel pressured or scorned for not choosing breastfeeding. The evidence does show that breastfeeding gives the best possible start in life, but we need to accept that for some of us, despite our best efforts, breastfeeding just isn't possible and that switching to formula doesn't make us a bad mother. Breastfeeding is not a competition; rather it is about providing maximum nutritional support for your baby, before solids are introduced.

THE BENEFITS OF BREASTFEEDING

Breastfeeding is encouraged by midwives and health visitors to sustain your baby's development and support your baby's future health. Some of these benefits include reducing your baby's risk of developing conditions such as eczema if you breastfeed exclusively for the first three months. It may also reduce the risk of your baby experiencing obesity or diabetes in later life.

Breastfeeding also has benefits for you. It has been shown to reduce the risk of breast cancer, ovarian cancer, osteoporosis and postnatal depression (see page 132), as well supporting the contraction of the uterus and healthy weight loss after pregnancy.

BOOSTING BREAST MILK PRODUCTION

Making breast milk is an energy-hungry process for your body and for this it needs the support of a healthy diet. During breastfeeding you will need to consume an extra 500 calories (100 calories more than you needed in your third trimester) per day for the first six months.

Eating a diet to support your blood sugar will support this milk production as well as your energy. When blood sugar drops too low (see page 24) from not following a balanced diet low in refined sugars or carbohydrates, not eating enough or leaving long gaps in between meals, eating will trigger stress hormones. This in turn reduces the production of hormones that initiate milk supply and the 'let-down' reflex when your baby is brought to the breast. Eat little and often, preferably three main meals and two snacks per day. Eating a wholesome breakfast will replenish your reduced stores of glucose from feeding at night. You will also need to make sure that you are drinking enough water, around 6–8 glasses a day and this can include herbal teas, such as peppermint or fennel.

It is thought that the diet you eat during breastfeeding is the first stage of weaning for your baby. The breast milk changes in flavour and consistency according to the foods that you eat – garlic, for example, has been found in breast milk just an hour after the mother consumed it.

WHY IS BREAST MILK SO GOOD?

The composition of breast milk changes considerably in the first week after birth. Initially you will produce colostrum, a protein-rich substance that is packed with antimicrobial properties and immune-enhancing factors. After the first few days, your milk will 'come in'. This can be an emotionally difficult time, so I advise you take good care of yourself and rest and eat well to support this period. This more mature milk will be a mixture of foremilk and hindmilk to support the hydration and growth of your baby. Nature is so clever and the consistency of your milk will change according to the climate, producing more foremilk (the more watery part) when the weather is hot to keep your baby well hydrated. This mature milk will also have higher amounts of growth factors, antibodies, white blood cells and other protective factors against infection.

Breast milk is also a melting pot of nutrients and healthy fats, including B vitamins, vitamins A and E, and the minerals calcium, iron, zinc and iodine. This 'nutrition soup' can give your baby all that is needed for healthy growth in the first six months of their life, as long as you too are feeding yourself well. After this period your baby will need food sources of zinc (see page 59) and iron (see page 59) that your breast milk may no longer be able to supply adequately.

In recent years, researchers have also discovered that breast milk contains cannabinoids. These compounds are thought to help protect your baby against viruses and harmful bacteria, protect the brain and the nervous system and have natural pain-relieving actions. They also stimulate hunger and healthy growth. In this natural state, cannabinoids are both protective and 'soothing' physically and mentally. The hormones oxytocin and prolactin produced by your body as you are feeding have been shown to moderate stress mechanisms in your baby. This, in combination with the natural cannabinoids, may explain why babies often feel calmer when feeding.

THE IMPORTANCE OF FAT IN BREASTFEEDING

Your diet can have a significant influence on the fat content of your milk. Eating plenty of good fats increases the fat percentage in your breast milk and therefore supports growth in your baby, and increases the supply of important enzymes for optimum digestion and absorption of nutrients. It will also support your baby's intake of fat-soluble nutrients such as vitamins A, D, E and K, as well as healthy cholesterol. This healthy cholesterol is critical for the formation of the brain and nervous system, as well as the strength of the digestive system. Eating trans fats (see page 41), however, can interrupt this and reduce the healthy fat content in breast milk so these are best avoided. Trans fats can be transferred through your breast milk.

A study conducted in Canada compared the breast milk of Canadian women with a 'typical' Western diet that included trans fats through commercial baked goods, margarine and fried foods, to the breast milk of Chinese women with a traditional diet that did not include these trans fats. The results showed a 33 times greater trans fats content in the breast milk of the Canadian women.

Your baby will rely on your consumption of omega-3 and omega-6 fats in your diet for the fatty acids DHA and EPA (see page 41). These fats remain as vital as they were in pregnancy for the healthy development of the brain and eyes. Following the guidelines on fats in pregnancy by eating eggs, nuts, seeds and their oils, and oily fish regularly can greatly support this. You may also benefit from taking an omega-3 supplement, especially if you do not like to eat fish.

The fatty acid CLA is another important fatty acid found in meat and dairy, which supports the development of your baby's immune system. In fact, CLA may be another factor that persuades you to choose organic in these foods sources. A Dutch study that looked at the breast milk of over 300 breastfeeding women found that the group that ate organic meat and dairy had a higher level of CLA than the women in the non-organic group.

YOUR KEY NUTRIENTS FOR BREASTFEEDING

The diet for healthy breastfeeding remains the same as that during pregnancy, but requires 500 more calories per day than your pre-pregnancy levels. If you have been eating a nourishing diet throughout your pregnancy your breast milk will be nutrient-rich. The Department of Health, however, recommends specific nutrients that are required in higher amounts during breastfeeding:

- **Vitamin A.** During breastfeeding your vitamin A requirement increases to 950 µg. This can be achieved by eating one sweet potato or an extra portion of carrots.
- **Vitamin B12.** This becomes even more important during the breastfeeding period, increasing from 1.6 µg to 2 µg daily. This can be done easily by eating an extra egg per day or having 4 g of yeast extract on your toast for example.
- **Vitamin D.** It is recommended that all breastfeeding mothers take a supplement containing 10 mg of vitamin D.
- **Zinc.** During breastfeeding you require around an extra 0.3 mg of zinc per day. This can be achieved from eating a small pot of yoghurt, sprinkling a tablespoon of pumpkin seeds on your porridge or eating a matchbox slice of cheese.
- **Calcium.** Calcium requirements increase considerably during lactation, almost doubling that needed in pregnancy. Around 250 mg of calcium is secreted into the breast milk per day. In order to prevent this being drawn from your bones, you need to be mindful of including calcium in your diet. You can do this by adding a cup of cooked greens to your meals, having a tablespoon of tahini on oatcakes or eating 25 g (1 oz) of hard cheese. See page 64 for calcium sources.
- **Omega-3.** It is recommended that women who are breastfeeding have a daily intake of at least 400 mg of the omega-3 fatty acid DHA per day. This is to support the development of your baby and your well-being too, as insufficient omega-3 fats have been shown to increase the risk of postnatal depression (see page 132). An intake of 400 mg daily is the equivalent of 2–3 portions of oily fish per week and, as the advice is to limit your intake of oily

fish to two portions a week during pregnancy and breastfeeding, taking an omega-3 supplement in addition to eating fish may be the most effective way for you to ensure you are getting enough DHA, especially if you are vegan or vegetarian.

- **Selenium.** Although this trace mineral is needed in small amounts, it becomes especially important during breastfeeding and needs to increase to 75 µg daily. This can be achieved by adding in 150 g/5 oz of wholegrain rice or snacking on as little as 10 g (½ oz) of brazil nuts a day.

BUT I DON'T HAVE THE TIME TO EAT WELL...

There are certain pearls of wisdom that should be passed on from mother to mother, some of which should definitely include practical tips on how to eat well when time is short but appetite is great. Getting into the habit of having snacks readily available for when you sit down to breastfeed is once of them. Find a comfy chair that you can hijack as your feeding chair for the next few months. Have a table by the side of it to put a large glass of water, a pot of mixed nuts/seeds or other healthy snack, a book or magazine and a radio. I often found juggling a baby and a book beyond my ability but listening to the radio was perfect company.

Another key tip is, at the start of each day, take a portion of your 'bulk cooking' out of the freezer in preparation for lunch or dinner. Or alternatively, throw ingredients into your slow cooker. In Chapter 14 I have laid out meal planners to support you during this 'fourth trimester', including ideas on where to find your extra 500 calories and healthy 'fast foods' (see page 164) for grabbing things in the moments when your baby sleeps.

Magnesium, vitamin B2 and iodine also remain important but don't need to be increased to meet the intake required during pregnancy. Your folate requirement (see page 49) reduces from 400 mg to 260 mg. Vitamin K also plays an essential role in blood-clotting and is produced by the healthy bacteria in the gut. However, at birth and in the early weeks of life your baby is not able to produce vitamin K as there is not sufficient beneficial bacteria to make it. Therefore eating plenty of these foods during breastfeeding can go some way to building up your baby's stores and healthy bacteria. These foods include broccoli, cabbage, cauliflower, peas and lentils.

WHAT ABOUT SUPPLEMENTS?

Supplements can support your intake of important nutrients for breastfeeding and recovery from birth, especially if you are vegan or vegetarian. However, a wholesome, nutritious diet as recommended in this book must be your starting point. The Department of Health recommends that all vegan breastfeeding mothers take a supplement of vitamin D and vitamin B12.

IMPROVING MILK SUPPLY

Your breast milk will naturally plateau at around three months and it is easy to think that your milk supply has diminished. In most cases, it is simply that your body and your baby have come into balance at this stage and supply is meeting demand, which makes the breasts feel less swollen. A group of herbs called galactagogues has been traditionally used to improve milk supply (and reduce it if there is an issue of oversupply) – these include fenugreek, ginger, caraway and blessed thistle. Adding fenugreek or caraway seeds and ginger into your cooking is a great way to boost milk supply. Seeds such as sunflower or sesame seeds, millet and almonds have also been used traditionally to improve breast milk supply, but for more specific support you may wish to seek the advice of a trained herbalist (see page 217).

WHAT IF I CAN'T BREASTFEED?

Breastfeeding doesn't come easily to all women. Sometimes a new mother may just need practical and emotional help with the technique. It is, however, a myth that all women are capable of breastfeeding – even in traditional cultures some women have not been able to breastfeed and relied on wet nurses. Some women are simply too unwell, unable to produce enough milk or may have a premature baby that has trouble latching on.

Many women who have their hearts set on breast-feeding become distraught at being unable to nurse their baby, as it is commonly believed to help with the bonding process. Whatever method of feeding you use, there is nothing to stop you bonding with your child and skin-to-skin contact is often recommended for mothers of premature babies who are unable to feed at the breast. What is most important is the love and care you give to your baby while you are feeding.

DOES STRESS AFFECT YOUR BREAST MILK?

Just like any other organ, the breasts are also affected by imbalances and lifestyle factors, such as stress. The release of stress hormones interrupts the production of prolactin, the hormone needed for efficient breast milk supply. Reducing your exposure to stress, whether it's turning your phone off, getting in some extra home help or asking for a relaxing massage from your partner, can help.

CAFFEINE AND ALCOHOL
DURING BREASTFEEDING

The current NHS guidelines on caffeine and alcohol intake when breastfeeding are very similar to those in pregnancy. Both caffeine and alcohol pass through the breast milk, can reduce milk supply and disrupt balanced blood sugar. They are also diuretics and increase the chances of dehydration.

When tiredness creeps in from broken sleep, you may feel drawn to have a strong cup of coffee. However, caffeine is stimulating to you and your baby and may interrupt your baby's ability to sleep deeply, so drink tea, coffee, green tea and other caffeine-containing foods no more than once or twice a day.

Alcohol affects the 'let-down' reflex as well as reducing how well the baby sucks. In fact, babies are thought to consume 30 per cent less milk in the first four hours after you've had your last alcoholic drink, but then compensate 8–16 hours afterwards by wanting to feed more. The presence of alcohol is strongest in the breast milk 30–60 minutes after drinking it, but will continue to affect your breast milk for several hours afterwards. The alcohol that you drink

'PUMP AND DUMP'?

There is a 'pump and dump' myth that you can pump your breast milk after drinking alcohol and discard it, but unless you are prepared to do this for all feeds within the next 12 hours, there really is no way to prevent the alcohol reaching your breast milk. So when breastfeeding, it's probably sensible to drink very little, for example, no more than one or two units (see page 82) once or twice a week. For more information, go to the NHS website (see page 214).

will go straight to your baby and will need to be processed by her liver which, as yet, will not have the liver enzymes necessary to do this. Having the odd glass of wine or champagne to celebrate is not going to be of harm, but I suggest that the majority of the time you avoid drinking alcohol when you are breastfeeding your baby.

CAN DIET HELP COLIC OR REFLUX?

Colic is defined as the uncontrollable crying that generally lasts for more than three hours a day, for at least three days a week and for three weeks. During a colic episode, your baby will mostly draw up her legs to her tummy and appear to be in pain. It usually starts to decline when your baby is around 10–12 weeks old.

Reflux, on the other hand, occurs when your baby's milk or food travel back up from the stomach along with stomach acid, into the oesophagus. She may also vomit (if she doesn't, it is known as 'silent reflux'). The defining nature of reflux tends to be the baby's desire to pull back and arch her back. This is usually the result of an immature sphincter between the oesophagus and the stomach, and tends to improve naturally as the baby grows.

Results from studies done on dietary influences on the development of colic and reflux are inconclusive. However, from my personal experience, and that of new mothers I've worked with, I know that some dietary changes can make a significant difference.

The most common triggers include eggs, soy, gluten-containing grains (wheat, barley, rye, spelt and Kamut), cow's milk, strawberries and chocolate. These foods need to be reduced with caution as many are also rich sources of the nutrients necessary to support healthy breast milk (for example, protein in cow's milk, and B vitamins and choline in eggs and grains). Different things affect different babies so just try eliminating one food at a time.

I would, however, advise you to seek the help of a trained nutritional therapist or speak to your health visitor before you start cutting out food groups, as sometimes changing the feeding position can be enough to reduce colic and reflux.

GOOD ALTERNATIVE FOOD SOURCES

- Gluten grains – substitute with millet, quinoa, buckwheat, amaranth, red rice or wild rice.
- Cow's milk – substitute with almond, rice and hemp milk. Some babies can tolerate goat's milk or sheep's products as the protein is less allergenic in these milks.
- Eggs – substitute with nuts or pulses for protein, iron and B vitamins.
- Caffeine – substitute with chicory coffee or redbush tea.
- Chocolate – substitute with carob chocolate.

Chamomile tea, lemon verbena tea, nettle tea and fennel tea can ease discomfort from wind and have anti-spasmodic properties for reducing cramps that can be associated with both colic and reflux. You can drink this yourself or add a couple of teaspoons of the cooled infusion to your baby's milk or to cooled boiled water. You may also want to investigate cranial osteopathy (see page 134) as this has been shown to benefit some babies if colic is influenced by structural issues, such as muscle tensions from the birth.

PROBIOTICS AND COLIC

If you are breastfeeding and your baby is experiencing colic or reflux, I recommend you try taking a probiotic supplement. There have been a number of recent studies that show a positive outcome on the baby's symptoms, such as reduced crying and fussing, when breastfeeding women have taken a probiotic that included a strain of flora called Lactobacillus reuteri.

Lactobacillus reuteri can also be found naturally in some fermented foods, such as the fermented milk drink kefir (see page 208) or fermented vegetables such as sauerkraut (see page 208) and kimchi, although go slowly with these as introducing too much in one go can leave you both feeling very windy.

COLIC OR REFLUX AND COW'S MILK

Colic may be due to lactose intolerance in some babies. A lactose intolerance means that your baby is sensitive to the lactose (a sugar) in the milk products that you are consuming, which is being passed down through your breast milk. This is primarily because of insufficient levels of the enzyme lactase that break this sugar down. This causes fermentation and the production of gases in your baby. Breast milk actually contains a low amount of lactose naturally, but because cow's milk is hydrogenated and pasteurised it can reduce the amount of other enzymes and proteins that work with your body to help break down lactose when we ingest it. Once you baby is 3–4 months old, she should be producing enough lactase enzyme to break down lactose on her own.

• • •

Breastfeeding can be one of the most profoundly intimate and loving exchanges between you and your baby. It can support a gentle transition from carrying your baby inside you and adjusting to the physical separateness that occurs naturally as a result of the birth. Take the time to listen and watch for your baby's cues in the early weeks. In time you will start to do this subconsciously and it will soon become a rhythmic, symbiotic process for you both. Eating the right diet throughout the breastfeeding months will provide maximum nourishment for you and your baby.

CHAPTER 13

NOURISHING YOUR BODY AND MIND WITH YOGA

Throughout the book I have focused on the importance of good nutrition for a healthy and happy pregnancy, but a healthy body is a healthy mind too. It is important to take a holistic approach to ensure that your levels of stress and anxiety are kept as low as possible and that you experience a general sense of well-being. This is not only important for you but for your baby, too. The bond between you and your baby is such that your emotional well-being can have an effect on everything from the pain you experience in labour to how well your child breastfeeds. Complementary therapies such as acupuncture and homeopathy, and gentle exercise such as yoga can help to reduce your levels of stress and anxiety, as well as prepare your body and mind for the hard work of labour.

THE BENEFITS OF PREGNANCY YOGA

During my pregnancies, I found immense support from a regular yoga practice working with experienced pregnancy yoga teacher Michelle Pearce (see page 219). Yoga during pregnancy, whether practised at home or in a group, can provide emotional and physical support and help prepare for birth. The rhythmic movements, gentle breathing practices, and the resonant sounds of yoga also offer ways of connecting with, and soothing, the unborn baby. Indeed the word yoga itself means 'to unite' and in pregnancy yoga this unity relates to that within the mother's body, mind and emotions, as well as that with her unborn baby.

Yoga can be enjoyed from the 12th week of pregnancy. When you go to a class, or sit on your yoga mat at home, you are primarily giving yourself *time* – time out from the normal demands of life, time to relax, and time to be with your baby. There are now plenty of pregnancy yoga DVDs and websites, such as YogaGlo (see page 219), that enable you to practise yoga in the comfort of your own home. However, you may find that going to a class offers you the chance to share your experiences of pregnancy and any concerns that you may have about giving birth with others who are on the same journey.

YOGA POSITIONS

Pregnancy yoga positions, or asanas, offer gentle ways for your body to relax, stretch and accommodate the changing weight of the baby. A good pregnancy yoga class should feel like a moving massage, with the whole body being invited to release stress and tension through a rhythmic series of movements. Standing, leaning, kneeling, being on all fours and being seated astride chairs are all commonly used positions in pregnancy yoga, and there are a wealth of books depicting these. If you are familiar with a range of positions, if you know what is comfortable for you and how to make full use of the supports around you – chairs, walls, cushions, other people! – you will have a good set of positions to choose from during birth.

It is important that your starting point for your pregnancy yoga is always with your *self*, with your body. Rather than simply following the instructions of a teacher or book, you must always ask yourself how the position or movement *feels*, whether it is right for you, or whether you would rather adjust it or find an alternative. This engagement with your pregnancy yoga practice lays the foundation stones for your engagement with delivery – if you are familiar with adjusting your position or your breathing to suit your needs during pregnancy, you will be primed to do the same during delivery.

BREATHING TECHNIQUES

A key element in pregnancy yoga is learning to watch the breath. This is normally done in a comfortable seated position with your eyes closed and by observing your breath, noticing when you are breathing in and when you are breathing out. You do not need to do anything more than this. The body knows how to breathe – your job is to do your best to remove tension from body and mind to enable yourself to breathe fully, easily and naturally. Saying affirmations works beautifully with these breathing techniques. For example, you might say the following to yourself as you breathe:

Breathing in I nourish my body,
and breathing out I relax.

From these simple beginnings, pregnancy yoga has built a rich variety of breathing practices designed to ensure a good supply of oxygen to your body and your baby, to quiet busy minds, still difficult emotions and to give birth. Sound can be added on the out-breath to focus the mind still further, and to bathe your body and baby in soothing vibrations. Practising sound work during pregnancy will also help you to feel comfortable making sounds during labour, which is an effective way of releasing strong sensations from the body.

EXPERIENCING STILLNESS

With its postures, breath-work, sound-work, affirmations and relaxation, pregnancy yoga offers a valuable space within which to rest inwardly with your baby. When the rhythmic movements of the asanas combine with simple breath awareness, and possibly sound or affirmation, you can experience the 'settling [of] the mind into stillness', which yoga guru Patanjali spoke of in his ancient Yoga Sutras. Within this stillness there is often great courage to be found, great acceptance, great peace, and the sense of surrendering to an incredible journey with unknown outcomes. Once the mind has quietened in this way, space arises, space in which the powerful voice of instinct can arise, arming you with the most valuable tool of all – the instinctive knowledge that your body knows just what to do.

10-MINUTE YOGA PRACTICE

Here Michelle has outlined a simple 10-minute yoga practice to support your mind and body during your pregnancy journey. Take time to become familiar with the different parts of this yoga sequence before trying to put it all together. Try the different positions, make any adjustments or omissions that feel right for you, and in this way make the individual asanas (postures) your own. If it feels good, it probably is good. If it feels uncomfortable, leave it out or adapt it so that it feels comfortable again.

The key is to use yoga practice as an opportunity for rest – to rest with yourself, your baby and your breath. It is a chance to undo and to build a place of quietness from which your baby will, in time, be born.

WHAT YOU WILL NEED
- Floor space
- Warmth – a light jumper and T-shirt perhaps
- Solitude
- Cushions
- 3–4 yoga blocks – these are a very worthwhile investment for pregnancy, birth and beyond.
- Gentle companion music if you wish
- A little time in your day

Note: You need to be 12 weeks or more into your pregnancy before doing this routine. Seek professional advice before exercising after this stage of pregnancy if you have any pregnancy complications.

STEP 1: MOVING MASSAGE

- Keep your eyes open
- Find a comfortable position
- Circle the hips in both directions – allow them to release
- Roll the shoulders back and feel the tension ease out of the muscles
- Shake out the hands and let go
- Open and stretch the jaw – yawn or sigh to release the tension if you need to
- Flex and extend the spine

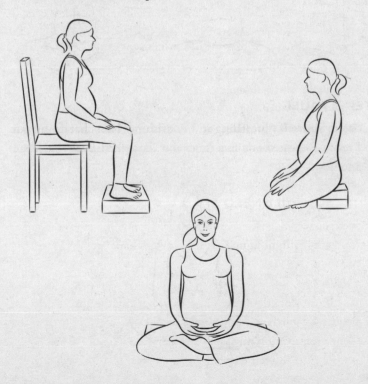

STEP 2: FIND THE BREATH

- Start with the hands in the prayer position at your heart
- Breathing in, take your hands above your head (if you have low blood pressure just raise your hands to shoulder height)
- Breathing out, let them float down to the sides and back to your heart centre
- Think of this as creating a bubble of light around you and your baby
- Repeat 3 times

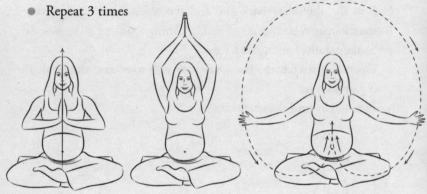

STEP 3: PAUSE

- Say to yourself, 'breathing in I nourish my baby, breathing out I relax.' Repeat slowly five times and allow the breath to deepen and slow.

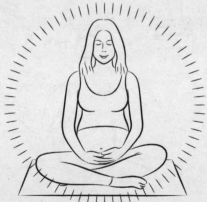

STEP 4: ALL FOURS STRETCH

- Fold a small blanket or use a pillow to cushion your right knee
- Move into an 'all fours' position
- Stretch out your left leg so that it is at a 90-degree angle
- Place the left knee on the ground and swap the blanket over to this knee.
- Stretch out your right leg so that it is at a 90-degree angle.
- You can repeat this process slowly twice more

Note: You may feel more comfortable leaning against a chair or wall for more stability.

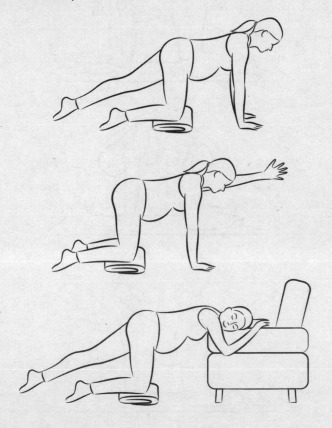

STEP 5: CAT POSE

- Position yourself on all fours
- Take a deep breath in
- As you let your breath go slowly, gently arch your back
- Wait in this position as you breathe in again
- As you breathe out, dip the back, only dipping the spine gently
- Continue this 4 or 5 times, finding a gentle, flowing rhythm

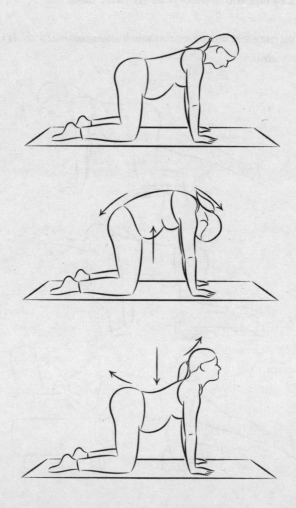

STEP 6: COMING UP TO STANDING

- Start on all fours
- Walk your hands back to your knees and press gently on the floor
- Use your knees to support you as you gently roll up through the spine
- Come all the way up to standing position
- Take a moment to find your feet and breathe here for a few moments
- As you get more confident, you may want to close your eyes

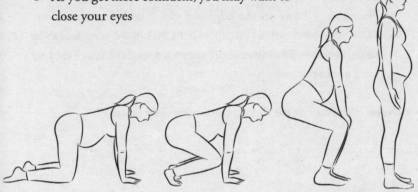

STEP 7: RELEASING THE HIPS

- Make sure your knees are soft
- Move your feet hip-distance apart
- Place your hands on your hips
- Roll your hips in an easy circle – imagine gently rocking your baby.
- After a minute, change direction

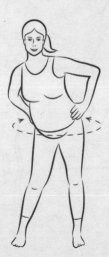

STEP 8: REST INTO SUPPORT

Rest your body in one of the supported positions:

- Lean your back and head flat against the wall with your feet slightly moved away and your knees softened. Rest for a minute or two
- Facing the wall, place your hands against the wall. Rest your forehead on the back of your hands. Place the top of your left foot close to the wall so your big toe is touching it. Soften your knee and rest
- Place your elbows on the edge of a chair, table or counter top. Place your forehead on your forearms and move your feet away so that you are leaning at right angles with a flat back. Rest here for a minute or two

Note: These can be excellent positions in early labour.

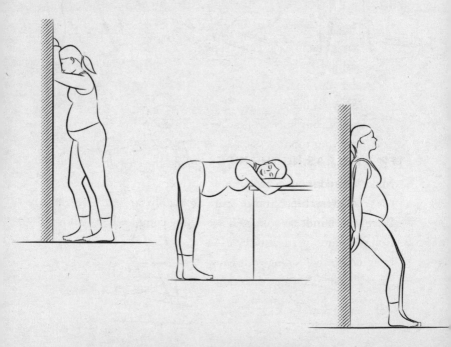

STEP 9: TIME TO BREATHE

- Make sure the base of your back is against the wall
- Place cushions beneath your knees and bottom if this makes it more comfortable for you
- Sit here with your hands resting on your belly and breathe, finding a gentle in and out breath rhythm
- As you breathe in, say to yourself, 'I nourish my baby' and as you breathe out, 'I relax'

STEP 10: LET GO

- Place a rug or blanket on the floor
- Lie down
- Place cushions
  - Under your head
  - Under your belly
  - Between your knees
  - Under your top foot
- Let your weight drop into the ground and the cushions beneath you more and more deeply
- Let go of everything, knowing you are totally safe and all is well
- Spend five minutes or longer here, feeling completely supported

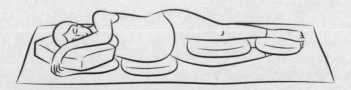

• • •

Nutrition plays a huge role in your healthfulness during pregnancy, but in order to experience nourishment on all levels, it is important that you look after your mental and emotional health too. A regular yoga practice during pregnancy can greatly complement a healthy diet and help to ensure that pregnancy and birth can be a happy and healthy experience.

CHAPTER 14

MEAL PLANNERS AND RECIPES

I know that a change in cooking style can leave you stuck for ideas of what to make, especially if you have not cooked with some of the recommended foods before.

This chapter provides menu plans and recipes to help you make your healthy pregnancy diet tasty and easy to follow. Most of the recipes can be prepared in advance, making them perfect to 'grab' in the smaller windows of time, such as when your baby is sleeping.

The very talented chef Sophie Wright, who has recently become a mother herself, has designed many of these recipes. She has therefore personally and professionally road-tested all these beautifully creative and nourishing meals.

There are also some great recipe books on the market and I have listed these in the Resources section (see page 220). Feel free to experiment with the recipes, swap things if they don't appeal, but keep up the variety.

SAMPLE DAILY MEAL PLANNERS

FIRST TRIMESTER

Breakfast Blueberry and Vanilla Crepes (see page 175)
Blackberry and Almond Compote (see page 171)

Lunch Tuna, Aduki Bean and Avocado Salad (see page 179)
Beetroot and Hazelnut Dip with crudités (see page 203)

Dinner   Mackerel with New Potato and Asparagus, Watercress and Almond Salad (see page 188)
Lamb, Coconut and Mango Pilau (see page 194)

SECOND TRIMESTER

Breakfast Quinoa Bircher with Blueberry Compote (see page 170)
Roasted Tomatoes on Rye with Avocado and Cottage Cheese (see page 174)

Lunch   Halloumi, Lentil and Roasted Pepper Salad with Rye Croutons (see page 181)
Brown Rice Kedgeree (see page 178)

Dinner   Slow-cooked Lamb with Preserved Lemons (see page 199)
Smoked Cod and Cannellini Beans (see page 193)

THIRD TRIMESTER

Breakfast Quinoa Porridge with Banana, Pear and Cinnamon (see page 173)
Coconut and Banana Bran Muffin (see page 169)

Lunch   Mackerel with Lemon and Potato Watercress Salad (see page 182)
Tofu, Spinach and Walnut Loaf (see page 185)

Dinner   Healthy Chicken and Sweet Potato Chips (see page 190)
Seafood Fish Pie with Cream Cheese Mash (see page 186)

Snack   Choose a snack from the 'instant energy-boosting snacks' list (see page 164) mid-afternoon

FOURTH TRIMESTER:
AFTER-BIRTH REGENERATION MENU

Breakfast Green Goodness Smoothie (see page 211)
With Poached Eggs and Steamed Chard on Sourdough (see page 176)
or
Chia Seed and Oat Breakfast Pots with Stewed Apple Compote (see page 172)

Lunch Beetroot, Orange and Ginger Soup (see page 177) with 5-minute Mackerel Pâté (see page 205) and Fennel and Flaxseed Oatcakes (see page 200)
Chicken, Root Vegetables and Rosemary Tray Bake (see page 198)

Dinner Lamb and Sweet Potato Hot Pot (see page 192)
Asian Sticky Pork Fillet with Steamed Asian Greens and Buckwheat Noodles (see page 196)

Snack Choose a snack from the 'instant energy-boosting snacks' list (see page 164) mid-afternoon

Drinks Hot water with freshly squeezed lemon juice and grated ginger
Warmed almond milk, heated in a pan with a cardamom pod, grated fresh cinnamon and a teaspoon of good-quality honey
Deeply Nourishing Spice Tea (see page 212)
Fortifying Mama Tea (see page 212)

HEALTHY 'FAST FOOD' OPTIONS

- Chia Seed and Oat Breakfast Pots with Stewed Apple Compote (see page 172)
- Quinoa Bircher with Blueberry Compote (see page 170)
- Coconut and Banana Bran Muffin (see page 169) with a small pot of plain live yoghurt
- Whole Earth baked beans or tinned tomatoes on wholemeal toast, with chopped parsley and grated Parmesan
- Chicken Broth (see page 207). Add a handful of shredded greens, such as spinach, and flaked cooked chicken
- Toasted bagel with ricotta cheese and quality smoked salmon
- Baked sweet potato with Creamy Spinach Dip (see page 203). Add a watercress or rocket salad, a tablespoon of sunflower seeds and olive oil dressing

INSTANT ENERGY-BOOSTING SNACKS

Add one of these snacks to support your extra daily calorie intake in the last trimester and two to reach your requirement in pregnancy:

- Grated carrot and houmus sandwich
- A dessertspoon of cashew, almond or peanut butter with apple segments
- Half an avocado with lemon juice and rock salt
- Shredded chicken with Beetroot and Hazelnut Dip (see page 203)
- Fennel and Flaxseed Oatcakes (see page 200) with Creamy Spinach Dip (see page 203)
- A slice of Nourish Bar (see page 210)
- A tablespoon of 5-Minute Mackerel Pâté (see page 205) with two Fennel and Flaxseed Oatcakes (see page 200)

- Miso soup with chopped shiitake mushrooms and shredded cabbage (add the mushrooms and cabbage into the bowl of boiling soup, place a lid on top and allow to sit for 5 minutes)
- Bowl of Chicken Broth (see page 207)
- Mixed nuts and seeds with Apple Chips (see page 204) or organic dried apricots
- Plain yoghurt with blueberries and flaked almonds
- Goat's cheese and sliced tomato on oatcakes
- Green Goodness Smoothie (see page 211)
- Tofu-Nut Balls (see page 206)
- Coconut and Banana Bran Muffin (see page 169)
- Parmesan Seeded Crispbreads (see page 201) with Beetroot and Hazelnut Dip (see page 203)

PLANNING AHEAD

I am the first to admit that during a working week or in the early stages of motherhood, preparing a full meal from scratch can, at times, be beyond our capabilities in both energy and time. One way to eat more healthy, home-cooked food is to plan ahead and 'bulk cook'. Now is a really good time to invest in a slow cooker or blender if you don't have one already. These two simple pieces of kitchen equipment can take a lot of the strain out of cooking. Throw your ingredients into a slow cooker in the morning (see the slow-cooked lamb recipe on page 194 for an example) and return from a day at work or a day with your baby to a warming, nourishing dinner. A blender can make light work of soups and smoothies, which can both provide quick and easy nourishment. Soups can be stored in the freezer.

When you are travelling or out for most of the day, you can avoid the need to grab high-sugar, high-fat and salty snacks by thinking ahead. Pack a slice of Nourish Bar (see page 210) or an apple and some oatcakes (see page 200) to support your energy and appetite. To help you plan ahead, you need a well-stocked cupboard.

YOUR NUTRITION IN PREGNANCY ESSENTIALS

Having a buoyant supply of healthy essentials in your kitchen cupboards will really help you to make healthy and nutritious choices throughout your pregnancy and in the early days of parenthood. Pre-booking regular online shopping slots can be a good reminder that you need to stock up.

Here I have listed those essential items that you will find invaluable when it comes to eating for a healthy pregnancy.

FOR THE CUPBOARD:

- Rice cakes
- Oatcakes
- Quinoa – whole and flaked
- Porridge oats
- Buckwheat or brown rice noodles
- Organic brown rice
- Dried organic apricots
- Dates
- Nut butter, such as cashew or almond
- Mixed nuts – walnuts, almonds and hazelnuts, for example – mix and keep in a sealed Mason jar
- Mixed seeds – sunflower, pumpkin and sesame, for example – mix and keep in a sealed Masons jar
- Tinned chickpeas or other pulses
- Lentils
- Whole Earth baked beans

FLAVOURINGS:

- Extra-virgin olive oil
- Coconut oil
- Apple cider vinegar

- Good-quality honey
- Miso
- Tamari or soy sauce
- Sea salt or rock salt
- Dried herbs, such as cumin, fennel seeds, turmeric, oregano and thyme
- Fresh root ginger
- Garlic
- Mustard
- Lemons

FRESH ESSENTIALS:

- Fresh herbs, such as coriander and parsley
- Avocado
- Apples
- Pears
- Eggs
- Plain yoghurt

FOR THE FREEZER:

- Bags of mixed berries
- Fish fillets
- Frozen peas
- Wholemeal bread or rye bread

Many of the recipes in this chapter can be made in advance and frozen. So, for example, you can pull out a healthy breakfast muffin the night before or a portion of soup in the morning for a quick lunch.

YOUR NUTRITION IN PREGNANCY SUPERFOOD CHART

Superfood	Rich source of
Quinoa	Magnesium, protein, fibre
Avocado	Folate, B vitamins, vitamin E
Brown rice	Folate, calcium, magnesium, zinc, iron, protein
Pumpkin seeds	Zinc, magnesium, protein, fibre
Sunflower seeds	Vitamin C, magnesium, protein, fibre
Almonds	Calcium, magnesium, zinc, folate, B vitamins, vitamin E, protein, fibre
Brazil nuts	Selenium, vitamin E, magnesium, protein, fibre
Eggs	Vitamin A, choline, vitamin B12, vitamin D, vitamin K, iron, selenium, iodine, protein
Green leafy vegetables	Folate, magnesium, vitamin C, fibre
Lentils	Folate, fibre, iron
Organic dried apricots	Iron, beta-carotene
Chicken broth	All minerals, essential amino acids, protein
Natural plain yoghurt	All B vitamins, calcium, magnesium, protein, beneficial flora

BREAKFASTS

COCONUT AND
BANANA BRAN MUFFIN

Rich in fibre, magnesium and potassium

Preparation time: 15 minutes
Cooking time: 20–25 minutes
Makes: 12 muffins

125 ml (4½ fl oz) coconut oil, melted
100 g (3½ oz) maple syrup
150 ml (5 fl oz) coconut milk
3 ripe bananas, mashed
2 free-range eggs
150 g (5 oz) wholemeal flour
125 g (4 oz) wheat bran
2 tsp baking powder
2 tsp ground cinnamon
2 tbsp desiccated coconut, plus 2 tsp to sprinkle over before baking

Preheat the oven to fan 180°C/350°F/Gas 4. Line a 12-hole muffin tray with muffin cases.

In a large bowl, mix together the oil, maple syrup, coconut milk, bananas and eggs. Whisk really well until all combined. In a separate bowl, mix the wholemeal flour with the bran, baking powder, cinnamon and coconut. Make a well in the centre. Pour in half of the wet mixture and combine well before mixing in the remainder. Spoon the mixture evenly into the muffin cases and sprinkle over the desiccated coconut.

Place the tray in the oven and cook for 20–25 minutes, until the muffins are golden and well risen. Remove from the oven and leave to cool before eating. You can store the muffins in an airtight container for up to 3 days or freeze them for up to 6 months; remove from the freezer and leave to defrost covered overnight to eat the next day.

Tip: These muffins are the perfect breakfast treat when you can't face a big breakfast.

QUINOA BIRCHER WITH BLUEBERRY COMPOTE

Rich in protein, fibre, potassium, magnesium, zinc, and vitamins B2 and B6

Preparation time: 5 minutes
Soaking time: overnight
Cooking time: 7–8 minutes
Serves: 2

75 g (2½ oz) quinoa flakes
75 g (2½ oz) pinhead or rolled oats
240 ml (8½ fl oz) almond or hazelnut milk
2 tbsp chia seeds
1 tsp ground cinnamon
zest of 1 large orange
2 tbsp chopped pistachios, plus extra to serve
1 apple or pear, grated with the skin on

Blueberry compote
100 g (3½ oz) blueberries
2 tbsp water
squeeze of lemon juice

To serve
2 tbsp natural yoghurt
1 tbsp pumpkin seeds

Place the flaked quinoa and oats into a large bowl and add the almond or hazelnut milk, chia seeds, cinnamon, orange zest, chopped pistachios and the grated apple or pear. Mix well and cover tightly with cling film. Leave in the fridge overnight where the mixture will absorb all the liquid.

To make the compote, place the blueberries into a small saucepan, and add the water and the lemon juice. Turn the heat on to a low simmer and cook for 5–6 minutes, until the blueberries start to burst and wilt. Simmer for a further 2 minutes, then remove from the heat and leave to cool in a small bowl.

When you are ready to serve, mix the quinoa bircher with the yoghurt and then layer it into bowls with the blueberry compote. Sprinkle over the extra chopped pistachios and some pumpkin seeds.

BLACKBERRY AND ALMOND COMPOTE

Rich in antioxidants, calcium and iron

Preparation time: 5 minutes
Cooking time: 10 minutes
Serves: 2

100 g (3½ oz) blackberries
½ tbsp honey
2 tbsp ground almonds

To serve
3 tbsp Greek or goat's yoghurt

Put the blackberries into a saucepan with a tablespoon of water and the honey. Cook over a low heat, stirring occasionally, for around 10 minutes until the berries have become soft and stewed in appearance. Add more water as it cooks, if necessary. Add the ground almonds, mix together and serve with Greek or goat's yoghurt.

CHIA SEED AND OAT BREAKFAST POTS WITH STEWED APPLE COMPOTE

Rich in omega-3, fibre, magnesium, potassium, and vitamins B, C and A

Preparation time: 5 minutes
Cooking time: 5 minutes
Soaking time: overnight
Serves: 2

100 g (3½ oz) pinhead oats
4 tbsp chia seeds
150 ml (5 fl oz) almond, hazelnut, organic cow's
    or rice milk (unsweetened)
zest of 1 orange
½ tsp ground cinnamon
2–3 tbsp good-quality runny honey

Apple compote
1 cooking apple, peeled and finely chopped
juice of ½ lemon
1 tbsp runny honey or agave syrup
pinch of ground cinnamon

To serve
runny honey
blueberries or pumpkin seeds

To make the compote, place the apple into a saucepan with the lemon juice and honey or agave syrup. Simmer for about 5 minutes, until the apple starts to break down. Add a little water if it is looking dry. Turn off the heat, stir in the cinnamon and leave to cool.

In a medium bowl, mix together the oats with the chia seeds, the milk of your choice, the orange zest, cinnamon and honey. Mix well, cover with cling film and leave to soak overnight in the fridge.

When ready to serve the next morning, layer the soaked chia seeds and oat mix with the apple compote. Add a final drizzle of honey and half a handful of pumpkin seeds or blueberries.

Tips:
- If you use a sweeter eating apple omit the honey.
- This breakfast is best made the night before to allow the chia seeds and oats to soak up all the milk. It also makes things much quicker and easier in the morning.

QUINOA PORRIDGE WITH BANANA, PEAR AND CINNAMON

Rich in vitamin B, zinc, iron, potassium and protein

Preparation time: 5 minutes
Cooking time: 25–30 minutes
Serves: 2

75 g (2½ oz) quinoa
200 ml (7 fl oz) almond milk or semi-skimmed milk
150 ml (5 fl oz) water
1 tsp ground cinnamon
2 tbsp manuka honey or other good-quality runny honey
1 pear, grated with the skin on
1 banana, mashed

To serve
1 tbsp pumpkin seeds
1 tbsp flaxseed

Wash the quinoa under cold water and transfer into a saucepan. Pour over the milk and water and place on the stove. Stir in the cinnamon. Bring the mxiture to the boil then turn down the heat and simmer for 15–20 minutes, stirring regularly so it does not stick to the bottom of the pan. Add the honey and stir well.

Continue to cook for another 5–10 minutes, until the quinoa is completely soft and has absorbed most of the liquid. Stir in the pear and banana. Serve in bowls with a sprinkling of the seeds on top.

ROASTED TOMATOES ON RYE WITH AVOCADO AND COTTAGE CHEESE

Rich in vitamin D, DHA, vitamin E, folate, vitamin B12, beta-carotene, selenium, vitamin C and protein

Preparation time: 15 minutes
Cooking time: 10 minutes
Serves: 2

10 baby plum tomatoes (on the vine are best)
olive oil
4 slices good-quality rye bread
1 ripe avocado
4 tbsp cottage cheese
zest and juice of ½ lemon
1 tbsp sunflower seeds
1 tbsp pumpkin seeds
1 tbsp avocado or hemp seed oil
sea salt and black pepper

Preheat the oven to fan 220°C/425°F/Gas 7. Place the tomatoes into a small baking dish and drizzle with a small amount of olive oil. Bake in the oven for 10 minutes until they start to burst.

Toast the rye bread. Cut the avocado in half and remove the stone. Scoop out the flesh with a large tablespoon and put it into a bowl. Mash with the back of a fork. Season with a small amount of sea salt and black pepper, and then fold in the cottage cheese. Stir in half of the lemon juice.

Pile the cottage cheese and avocado mixture on top of the toast. Sprinkle over the lemon zest and seeds. Add the roasted tomatoes and drizzle with the avocado or hemp oil and the remaining lemon juice.

BLUEBERRY AND VANILLA CREPES

Vitamin C, fibre, calcium and manganese

Preparation time: 10 minutes
Cooking time: 25–30 minutes
Makes: 6–8 crepes

150 g (5 oz) wholemeal or spelt flour
1 large free-range egg
325 ml (11½ fl oz) almond or semi-skimmed milk
20 g (¾ oz) butter
50 ml (2 fl oz) rapeseed oil for cooking the crepes

For the filling
200 g (7 oz) ricotta cheese
4 tbsp good-quality runny honey
1 vanilla pod, split lengthways and seeds removed,
*   or 1 tsp vanilla bean paste*
zest of 1 orange

Warm blueberries
200 g (7 oz) blueberries
2 tbsp water
1 tbsp good-quality runny honey or agave syrup

Make your crepe batter by sifting the flour into a large bowl. Create a well in the centre and crack in the egg. Pour in half of the milk. Using a whisk, mix well, incorporating the flour from the sides of the bowl bit by bit. Once you have formed a thick paste, add the remaining milk and whisk again until smooth. Leave the batter to rest while you make your filling.

In a medium bowl, combine the ricotta with the honey, vanilla and orange zest, and beat well. Place the blueberries into a small saucepan with the water and honey or agave, and turn the heat to low. Cook for 5–6 minutes or until the blueberries start to wilt a little. Turn the heat off but cover the pan to keep warm.

Heat a 15 cm (6 in) non-stick frying pan, or crepe pan if you have one, and add the butter. Once melted, pour the butter into the crepe batter and whisk to combine. Heat a little of the oil in the same pan and, once hot, add a ladle of the crepe mixture. Swirl the pan around as soon as the mixture hits the hot oil to make sure the whole base of the pan is covered. Place the pan back on the heat and cook for 2 minutes before flipping the crepe over and cooking the other side for around 1 minute. Remove from the pan on to a plate and keep warm while you make the remaining crepes.

Lay your warm crepes out one at a time and fill with a little of the ricotta mixture before rolling up into 'cigars' and serving with a couple of spoonfuls of the blueberries.

POACHED EGGS AND STEAMED CHARD ON SOURDOUGH

Rich in choline, iodine, iron, vitamin B12, magnesium, zinc and protein

Preparation time: 5 minutes
Cooking time: 10 minutes
Serves: 1

1 free-range egg
50g (2 oz) Chard
1 tsp white wine vinegar
1 tbsp olive oil

1 slice of sourdough bread
sea salt and black pepper

Pour 500 ml (17½ fl oz) of water into a saucepan with the vinegar. Bring to the boil.

While the water is coming to the boil, place the chard into a steamer and steam for 3 minutes or until just wilted. Strain the greens, transfer to a bowl and add the olive oil, a pinch of salt and black pepper, and leave to one side while you cook the egg.

Once the water and vinegar have boiled, bring the water down to a simmer. Carefully break the egg into the water and leave to cook at a gentle simmer for 5 minutes.

While the egg is cooking, toast your slice of sourdough.

When the toast is done, top with the greens, and add your egg by removing it from the water with a slotted spoon.

You can replace the sourdough with rye or wholemeal bread, or substitute the chard for any greens, such as spinach or kale, to suit your tastes or the season.

LUNCH

BEETROOT, ORANGE AND GINGER SOUP

Rich in fibre, iron, vitamin C, beta-carotene, magnesium and gingerols

Preparation time: 10 minutes
Cooking time: 30 minutes
Serves: 2

1 tbsp rapeseed or coconut oil
1 onion, chopped

1 medium potato
2½ cm (1 in) piece of fresh ginger, grated or finely chopped
zest of 1 orange
juice of 2 oranges
3 medium beetroots, boiled or roasted, and diced
1.2 litres (2 pints) chicken or vegetable stock (preferably fresh)
natural yoghurt
sea salt and freshly ground black pepper

Heat the oil in a large, heavy-based sauce pan, add the onion and fry over a gentle heat for about 5 minutes or until soft. Add the potato and ginger and fry for 3 minutes. Add most of the orange zest, and the orange juice, beetroot and stock, and bring to the boil. Simmer for about 20 minutes or until the potato is tender. Transfer the soup to a blender and blitz until smooth. Season to taste, then pour the soup into bowls. Garnish with the remaining orange zest and a swirl of natural yoghurt.

BROWN RICE KEDGEREE

Rich in omega-3, vitamins B12, B3, B1, B2, folic acid, iron, magnesium, calcium, fibre and protein

Preparation time: 5 minutes
Cooking time: 45 minutes
Serves: 2

350 g (12 oz) undyed smoked haddock
1 tbsp coconut oil
1 small onion, finely chopped
1 tsp curry powder
½ tsp turmeric
90 g (3¼ oz) brown rice, rinsed
1 tbsp tomato purée

125 g (4 oz) spinach leaves
2 tbsp goat's yoghurt (optional)
2 hard-boiled eggs, quartered
sea salt and black pepper

Bring 600 ml (1 pint) of water to the boil in a large, high-sided frying pan. Reduce the heat, add the smoked haddock and simmer for 3–4 minutes, until just cooked. Transfer the fish to a plate, strain the cooking liquid into a bowl and set aside.

Heat the oil in a large lidded saucepan, add the onion and cook over a medium heat for 2–3 minutes. Sprinkle in the curry powder and turmeric, and cook for another 2 minutes.

Stir in the rice and tomato purée, then pour in the reserved cooking liquid and bring to the boil. Reduce the heat, cover and simmer for 40–50 minutes until the rice is tender, stirring in the spinach just before the rice is cooked.

Meanwhile, remove and discard the skin and any bones from the haddock and separate the flesh into flakes.

Stir the yoghurt into the rice, add salt and pepper to taste, then gently mix in the flaked haddock. Spoon on to a warm serving dish, arrange the eggs on the rice and serve with steamed kale.

TUNA, ADUKI BEAN AND AVOCADO SALAD

Rich in selenium, iron, folate, omega-3, magnesium, potassium, fibre and vitamin E

Preparation time: 15 minutes
Cooking time: 6–10 minutes
Serves: 2

2 x 125 g (4 oz) tuna steaks
rapeseed oil

juice of ½ lemon
sea salt and black pepper

Salad

1 tin aduki beans, drained weight (approx. 200 g/7 oz)
1 ripe avocado, chopped into 1–2 cm (½–¾ in) pieces
1 celery stick, finely chopped
2 handfuls of cooked kale
25 g (1 oz) flat-leaf parsley, finely chopped
1 tbsp pumpkin seeds

Dressing

2 tsp Dijon mustard
juice of ½ lemon
1 tbsp apple cider vinegar
3 tsp rapeseed oil

Season the tuna steaks on both sides with salt and pepper, and drizzle with a little rapeseed oil. Heat a griddle pan and cook the tuna steaks for 3 minutes on each side, or slightly longer if you prefer them well done. Squeeze over the lemon juice, remove the steaks from the pan and leave them to rest.

Combine all the salad ingredients in a large bowl. Make the dressing by putting all the ingredients into a small jar. Place the lid on and shake well. Once the dressing has emulsified, toss three quarters of it into the salad.

Serve the salad with the sliced tuna steak on top and pour over the remaining dressing.

Tip: This dish can also be made with tinned tuna. It is a really simple salad for an easy lunch at home or to take to work.

HALLOUMI, LENTIL AND ROASTED PEPPER SALAD WITH RYE CROUTONS

Rich in potassium, magnesium, phytoestrogens, protein, beta-carotene, vitamin C, folic acid, calcium and iron

Preparation time: 15 minutes
Cooking time: 20–25 minutes
Serves: 2

100 g (3½ oz) uncooked Puy lentils, or 200 g (7 oz) tinned or ready-to-eat
rapeseed oil
2 garlic cloves, squashed but not peeled
2 slices stale rye bread, or any other wholemeal or seeded bread
150 g (5 oz) halloumi cheese, cut into 2½ cm (1 in) pieces
12–15 ripe baby plum tomatoes, halved
2 large roasted red peppers, sliced
2–3 large handfuls of baby watercress
sea salt and black pepper

Dressing
2 tsp Dijon mustard
2 tbsp sherry vinegar
3 tbsp rapeseed oil
sea salt and black pepper

If you need to cook the lentils, do this first. Wash them in cold water until the water runs clear. Transfer the drained lentils to a saucepan and add enough water to cover the lentils by 2½ cm (1 in). Place the pan over a high heat and bring the water to the boil, then turn down the heat and allow to simmer for 10–15 minutes, until the lentils are tender. Once cooked, drain, transfer the lentils to a bowl and season with a little salt.

Now make the dressing. Combine all the dressing ingredients in a small jar, season and put the lid on. Shake well until the dressing has combined and emulsified. Pour half over the warm lentils.

Heat a large frying pan and add 2 dessertspoons of rapeseed oil. Add the squashed garlic and tear in the stale bite-size pieces of of bread to make croutons. Toast the bread in the hot oil for 5–6 minutes, turning the pieces over halfway through until they are golden brown. Remove the croutons from the pan and leave them to drain on a piece of kitchen towel. Add a little more oil to the pan and fry the halloumi. Cook for 2–3 minutes or until the pieces turn slightly golden. Now add the tomatoes and the peppers. Heat through for 2–3 minutes before stirring in the lentils.

Place the watercress into a large serving bowl and spoon over the hot lentil mixture. Season with pepper and pour over the remaining dressing. Top with the toasted croutons before tossing well. Serve while it's still warm.

Tip: I buy my red peppers ready roasted in a jar for convenience.

MACKEREL WITH LEMON AND WATERCRESS POTATO SALAD

Rich in omega-3, vitamin D, fibre and folate

Preparation time: 10 minutes
Cooking time: 20 minutes
Serves: 2

1 tbsp rapeseed oil
2 mackerel fillets
sea salt and black pepper

Potato salad
200 g (7 oz) new potatoes, washed
2 tbsp crème fraîche
2 tsp baby capers

zest of 1 lemon and juice of ½ lemon
1 tsp horseradish cream or wholegrain mustard
2 handfuls of watercress, roughly chopped
sea salt and black pepper

To make the potato salad, put the potatoes into a saucepan and cover with boiling water from the kettle. Add a pinch of salt and place over a high heat. Boil for about 15 minutes, depending on the size of the potatoes, until cooked through. Once cooked, drain well and cut each potato in half or into three, depending on their size, so all the pieces are roughly equal. Put the potato pieces into a large bowl and add all the remaining salad ingredients, except the watercress and half the lemon juice. Season well and leave to one side. It's best to do this while the potatoes are still hot to allow all the flavours to infuse.

Heat a frying pan on the highest heat and pour in the rapeseed oil. Season the mackerel with salt and pepper. When the pan is hot, place the mackerel in the pan skin side down. Press the fish flat into the pan with a spatula to prevent it curling. Cook for 4 minutes on the skin side before flipping it over and cooking for another 2 minutes. Turn off the heat.

Add the watercress to the still-warm potatoes and pile the salad on to your plates. Top with the mackerel and serve with the remaining lemon juice.

SMOKED SALMON AND CREAM CHEESE MINI FRITTATAS

Rich in omega-3, calcium, protein, vitamins B6 and B12

Preparation time: 15 minutes
Cooking time: 15 minutes
Makes: 12

flavourless oil, such as sunflower or groundnut for greasing
8 large free-range eggs
50 ml (2 fl oz) milk
100 g (3½ oz) low-fat cream cheese
zest of 2 lemons
15 g (½ oz) dill, chopped
150 g (5 oz) smoked salmon, chopped
25 g (1 oz) grated Parmesan
sea salt and black pepper

Preheat the oven to fan 180°C, 350°F, Gas 4. Take a 12-hole muffin tin and grease each hole with a little oil. Cut out 12 small squares (approximately 10 x 10 cm/4 x 4 in) of parchment paper and push each one into a muffin hole. You should have a little overhang in each hole.

Crack the eggs into a bowl and whisk well. Add the milk and half the cream cheese and whisk again. Stir in the salt and pepper, lemon zest and dill and three quarters of the smoked salmon. Pour the mixture evenly into each muffin hole. Add a teaspoon of the remaining cream cheese into the centre of each frittata. Top with the remaining salmon. Grate the Parmesan over each frittata and cook in the oven for 15 minutes, until the frittatas are set and slightly spongy to the touch.

Remove the frittatas from the tray and leave to cool before serving.

Tip: These frittatas are a really good staple to have in your fridge for when you don't have time to make yourself a full meal.

TOFU, SPINACH AND WALNUT LOAF

Rich in protein, folate, iron, omega-3 and magnesium

Preparation time: 20 minutes
Cooking time: 1 hour 20 minutes
Serves: 4–5

oil for greasing
1 tbsp nut oil
1 onion, chopped
450 g (1 lb) mushrooms, very finely chopped
6 large garlic cloves, minced
125 g (4 oz) ground walnuts
900 g (2 lb) spinach, chopped, or frozen spinach
2 tbsp Worcestershire sauce
1 tsp sea salt
1 tbsp tamari (wheat-free soy sauce)
450 g (1 lb) firm tofu, mashed
170 g (6 oz) brown rice
freshly ground black pepper
¼ tsp ground nutmeg
horseradish sauce to serve
paprika to serve

Preheat the oven to fan 180°C/350°F/Gas 4. Lightly oil a medium loaf tin.

Heat the nut oil in a deep frying pan. Add the onion, mushrooms, and garlic, and sauté over a medium heat for about 8–10 minutes

Add the walnuts, spinach, Worcestershire sauce and salt. Stir and cook for another 5–8 minutes, or until the spinach is wilted and everything is well mixed. Turn off the heat.

Stir in the tamari, tofu, rice, black pepper and nutmeg. When everything is thoroughly combined, taste to adjust seasonings. Pour the mixture into the prepared loaf tin, and bake uncovered for 1 hour. Allow the loaf to rest for about 10 minutes before serving. Serve hot, with horseradish sauce and a sprinkling of paprika.

DINNER

SEAFOOD FISH PIE WITH CREAM CHEESE MASH

Rich in omega-3, selenium, iodine, vitamin B12 and zinc

Preparation time: 40 minutes

Cooking time: 55 minutes

Makes: 4–6 individual pies

2 tbsp rapeseed oil
3 shallots, finally chopped
1 bay leaf
125 ml (4½ fl oz) white wine
200 ml (7 fl oz) fish stock
200 g (7 oz) low-fat cream cheese
200 g (7 oz) salmon, skinned and diced into 2 cm (¾ in) chunks
200 g (7 oz) undyed smoked haddock, skinned and diced into 2 cm
  (¾ in) chunks
125 g (4 oz) peeled raw tiger prawns
125 g (4 oz) mussels, cooked and removed from their shells
2 handfuls of petits pois
125 g (4 oz) broccoli florets
juice and zest of 1 lemon
15 g (½ oz) chopped parsley
sea salt and black pepper

Topping

1 kg (23 oz) Maris Piper potatoes
100 g (3½ oz) low-fat cream cheese
50 g (2 oz) Parmesan, grated
sea salt

To serve

steamed kale or spring greens

Preheat the oven to fan 180°C/350°F/Gas 4. Heat the rapeseed oil in a large saucepan and add the shallots and bay leaf. Fry over a medium heat for 5–6 minutes or until the shallots are translucent; don't allow them to burn. Add the white wine, fish stock and cream cheese. Simmer for about 15 minutes or until the mixture has thickened and reduced by a third. All the alcohol will have evaporated off at this point, leaving you with a non-alcoholic, but delicious sauce.

Now add in the fish, seafood, petits pois and broccoli. Stir well and season with salt, lots of pepper and the lemon juice and zest. Add the chopped parsley and turn off the heat. Spoon the mixture into 4–6 individual pie dishes and leave to cool.

Meanwhile, peel all the potatoes and cut them into large pieces. Place them into a saucepan of cold salted water and bring to the boil. Cook until tender – around 15 minutes should be long enough.

Remove the potatoes from the heat and drain. Leave them to stand for 5–10 minutes to allow some of the excess moisture to evaporate.

Mash the potatoes either with a masher or pass them through a potato ricer. Add the cream cheese and season with a little salt. Top each of your pies with the mash and spike the tops using a fork, to achieve a nice crispy top. Grate over the Parmesan and bake in the oven for 35 minutes, until golden brown and bubbling. Serve with steamed kale or spring greens.

MACKEREL WITH NEW POTATO AND ASPARAGUS, WATERCRESS AND ALMOND SALAD

Rich in magnesium, beta-carotene, iron, fibre, and vitamins B6, D and K

Preparation time: 10 minutes

Cooking time: 20 minutes

Serves: 2

10 whole new potatoes, scrubbed and washed but not peeled

2 mackerel fillets

1 tbsp rapeseed oil

12 spears asparagus, woody ends removed but not peeled

2–3 handfuls of watercress

2–3 tbsp toasted flaked almonds

25 g (1 oz) parsley, roughly chopped

Dressing

2 tbsp crème fraîche

juice and zest of 1 lemon

2 tsp wholegrain mustard

sea salt and black pepper

Preheat the grill. Cook the potatoes in boiling salted water for 12–15 minutes or until tender. While the potatoes are cooking, lay the mackerel fillets skin side up on a baking tray and rub them with the oil. Place the tray under the hot grill and cook for 7 minutes. Once cooked through, turn off the heat and allow to rest.

Drain the cooked potatoes and cut them in half or quarters depending on their size. Steam the asparagus for 2–3 minutes until just tender and still al dente.

Place the warm potatoes, asparagus, watercress, almonds and parsley into a large bowl and mix well.

Make the dressing by mixing the crème fraîche with the lemon zest and most of the lemon juice and the mustard. Season with salt and pepper before mixing through the salad.

Serve the salad on a big platter and lay the mackerel fillets on top, and give a final squeeze of lemon juice.

Tips:

- This dish is also great with smoked mackerel fillets if you can get them fresh.
- Leaving the new potatoes whole when you cook them retains more of the nutrients.

PUMPKIN CHEESY RAVIOLI BAKE WITH SAGE

Rich in beta-carotene, calcium, and vitamins K and D

Preparation time: 15 minutes
Cooking time: 45 minutes
Serves: 4–6

*400 g (14 oz) pumpkin or butternut squash, unpeeled and cut into
   thin slices or thin wedges*
1 tbsp good-quality runny honey
2 tbsp rapeseed oil
6–8 sage leaves
200 g (7 oz) cream cheese
125 g (4 oz) mozzarella
50 g (2 oz) Parmesan, grated
1 tbsp Dijon mustard
550g (1lb 3½ oz) fresh spinach and ricotta ravioli
sea salt and black pepper

To serve
baby leaf spinach

Preheat the oven to fan 190°C/375°F/Gas 4. Coat the pumpkin or butternut squash in the honey and rapeseed oil by tossing them together in a large bowl. Add the sage leaves and season with salt and pepper.

Melt the cream cheese in a saucepan over a gentle heat, then add the mozzarella, half of the Parmesan and the mustard. Continue to heat, stirring frequently, until all the cheese has melted.

Place the uncooked fresh ravioli in a large baking dish and pour over the cheese sauce. Mix well. Lay the sliced pumpkin or butternut squash and sage leaves on top (the sage leaves will crisp up while cooking). Have some of the pumpkin poking upwards and overlapping so it will brown and caramelise in places. Scatter over the remaining Parmesan.

Cook in the oven for 35 minutes, until the pumpkin is caramelised and tender, and the cheese sauce is bubbling. Remove from the oven and allow to cool slightly before serving with a baby leaf spinach salad for extra iron.

HEALTHY CHICKEN AND SWEET POTATO CHIPS

Rich in vitamin B6, beta-carotene, vitamin C, carbohydrate, selenium and protein

Preparation time: 30 minutes
Cooking time: 30 minutes
Serves: 2

2 free-range chicken breasts, skin removed
100 ml (3½ fl oz) buttermilk
sea salt and black pepper

For the coating
2 slices stale wholewheat bread
50 g (2 oz) bran flakes

2 tbsp chopped parsley
sea salt and black pepper

Sweet potato chips
2 large sweet potatoes, washed but not peeled
½ tsp smoked paprika
½ tsp ground cumin
½ tsp dried oregano
2 tbsp rapeseed oil
sea salt and black pepper

Preheat the oven to fan 190°C/375°F/Gas 5. Start by marinating the chicken. Pour the buttermilk into a large bowl and season with salt and pepper. Butterfly the chicken breasts by cutting them in half lengthways and opening them out like a book. Place the chicken into the buttermilk, cover and leave to marinade and tenderise for 20 minutes while you prepare the chips and breadcrumbs.

Cut the sweet potatoes into 3 cm- (1¼ in-) thick chips and place into a bowl. Leave the skin on as this not only tastes delicious but it will also stop the chips from falling apart during cooking. Sprinkle over the paprika, cumin and oregano, and season with salt and pepper. Add the oil and toss everything together to coat the chips. Line a baking tray with non-stick baking parchment and lay on the seasoned chips.

Make the chicken coating by blitzing the stale bread with the bran flakes in a food processor until you have fine breadcrumbs. Add in the chopped parsley. Remove the chicken from the buttermilk and coat each piece well in all the breadcrumbs.

Place the chicken on to the tray with the chips and put it into the oven. Cook for 15 minutes, then turn everything over and cook for another 15 minuntes.

Once the chips are crispy on the outside and the chicken is nice and golden, remove from the oven and serve with a wedge of lemon and a sprinkle of salt.

LAMB AND SWEET POTATO HOT POT

Rich in beta-carotene, zinc, protein, and vitamins C and B12

Preparation time: 20 minutes

Cooking time: 1 hour 10 minutes

Serves: 4

4 tbsp rapeseed oil

800 g (1 lb 12 oz) grass-fed lamb neck fillets, diced

350 g (12 oz) white onions, sliced

2 garlic cloves, chopped

1 tbsp Worcestershire sauce

1 tbsp thyme leaves

450 ml (16 fl oz) lamb or beef stock

800 g (1 lb 12 oz) sweet potatoes, peeled and thinly sliced

25 g (1 oz) butter

2 tbsp grated Parmesan

sea salt and black pepper

To serve

spring greens

Preheat the oven to fan 190°C/375°F/Gas 4. Place an ovenproof casserole dish that has a tight-fitting lid on the hob and add 2 tablespoons of rapeseed oil. Turn the heat up high and when the oil is hot, add the diced lamb; you will probably need to cook the lamb in two batches to seal the meat evenly. Cook the first batch for 5–6 minutes, only turning the lamb over once it has browned and caramelised. Season well with salt and pepper as you go. Remove the sealed lamb from the dish and leave to one side on a plate while you repeat the process with the second batch.

Once all the lamb has been sealed and removed from the dish, add the remaining oil and the onions. Cook for 6–8 minutes until soft and translucent, before adding the garlic, Worcestershire sauce and thyme leaves. Cook for a further 2 minutes. Remove the onion mixture from the pan and set aside with the lamb.

While the dish is still hot on the stove, add 2–3 tablespoons of the stock and deglaze, scraping any toasted bits from the bottom of the dish. Turn off the heat. In a separate saucepan heat the remaining stock. Add the first layer of sweet potatoes. Spread over a little of the cooked onion mixture and the sealed lamb before adding another layer of sweet potatoes to the bottom of the casserole dish. Repeat the process, finishing with a neat layer of sweet potatoes. Pour over all the hot stock.

Melt the butter in a small saucepan or the microwave. Brush the top of the Hot Pot with the melted butter and sprinkle over the Parmesan. Put the lid on the dish and cook in the oven for 50 minutes. Remove the lid after 30 minutes to allow the top to brown. Serve with steamed spring greens.

SMOKED COD AND CANNELLINI BEANS

Rich in folate, iron, fibre, selenium and vitamin B12

Preparation time: 10 minutes
Cooking time: 15 minutes
Serves: 2

1 tbsp rapeseed oil or ghee
1 large white onion, sliced
100 ml (3½ fl oz) white wine
200 ml (7 fl oz) fish stock or vegetable stock
1 bay leaf
400 g (14 oz) undyed smoked cod or haddock, skinned
2 x 400 g (14 oz) tin cannellini beans, drained
25 g (1 oz) parsley, chopped
15 g (½ oz) chives, chopped

2 tbsp half-fat crème fraîche
sea salt and black pepper

To serve
2 lemon wedges
2 slices crusty wholemeal, spelt or seeded bread

Heat the oil in a large high-sided frying pan and add the sliced onion. Fry for 5–6 minutes until it is soft and slightly translucent. Pour the wine and stock into the pan and add the bay leaf – the alcohol will evaporate off during cooking. Lay the skinless fish in the pan and bring the liquid to the boil. Once boiling, turn the heat right down and leave to simmer for 2–3 minutes. When the fish starts to flake easily, remove it from the cooking liquor and set aside. Remove the bay leaf and discard it, and turn off the heat.

Pour away half of the cooking liquor and reserve the other half in the pan, along with the onions. Turn the heat back on and add the cannellini beans to pan. Boil for 3–4 minutes until the liquid starts to thicken, then flake in the cooked fish, along with the chopped herbs and the crème fraîche. Season well and serve with a wedge of lemon and some crusty bread.

Tip: The crème fraîche can be replaced with mascarpone.

LAMB, COCONUT AND MANGO PILAU

Rich in magnesium, selenium, zinc, beta-carotene, vitamin B and vitamin C

Preparation time: 20 minutes
Cooking time: 1 hour 40 minutes
Serves: 2

2 tbsp rapeseed oil
200 g (7 oz) lamb neck fillet, diced, preferably grass-fed

1 large white onion, sliced
1 garlic clove, sliced
5 cm (2 in) ginger, grated
1 large chilli, finely chopped
2 tsp ground cumin
2 tsp ground coriander
pinch of saffron
4 cardamom pods, squashed
450 ml (16 fl oz) lamb or chicken stock
200 ml (7 fl oz) coconut milk
200 g (7 oz) brown rice, washed

To serve
1 large ripe mango, diced
½ red chilli, chopped
25 g (1 oz) coriander, chopped
juice and zest of 1 lime

Preheat the oven to fan 180°C/350°F/Gas 4 if you want to cook this in the oven; you can also cook this on the hob or in a slow cooker. Place a large lidded casserole dish on the stove and turn the heat up high. Pour in the oil and, when hot, add the lamb. Seal the lamb in the oil for about 5–6 minutes, until golden on all sides. Once browned, removed the lamb from the pan and add the onion. Fry for 4–5 minutes until it starts to colour slightly, then add the garlic, ginger and all the spices. Cook for a few minutes more, then return the lamb to the dish, along with the stock and coconut milk. Put the lid on, reduce the heat and simmer for 1 hour on the hob or cook in the oven for 1 hour. Alternatively, transfer everything to a slow cooker and cook for 2–3 hours, until the meat is tender.

Add the rice to the dish and stir well. Replace the lid and cook for a further 30 minutes, or until the rice is lovely and tender if using a slow cooker. While the rice is cooking, make the mango salad. Mix the mango with the chilli, coriander, and the lime juice and zest in a bowl. Serve the lamb and rice straight from the pot, with the mango salsa on top.

ASIAN STICKY PORK FILLET WITH STEAMED ASIAN GREENS AND BUCKWHEAT NOODLES

Rich in Co-enzyme Q10, vitamin B (especially B12), vitamin E, potassium, magnesium and manganese

Preparation time: 30 minutes
Cooking time: 30–40 minutes
Serves: 4

1 x 350–400 g (12–14 oz) pork fillet
2 tbsp sesame seeds, toasted, plus extra to serve

Marinade
2 tbsp rice wine vinegar
6 tbsp dark soy sauce
1 tsp cornflour
5 cm (2 in) piece of fresh ginger, grated
3 garlic cloves, grated
2 tsp chilli paste or large pinch of chilli flakes
3 tbsp runny honey
2 tsp toasted sesame seed oil

Greens and noodles
300 g (10½ oz) buckwheat noodles
2 tbsp rapeseed oil
2½ cm (1 in) piece of fresh ginger, cut into matchsticks
2 garlic cloves, peeled and thinly sliced

300 g (10½ oz) Asian greens, such as pak choi and Chinese cabbage,
   trimmed
juice of 1 lime
2 tbsp light soy sauce
toasted sesame seed oil

Preheat the oven to fan 180°C/350°F/Gas 4. Make the marinade by combining all the ingredients well in a large bowl. Coat the pork fillet in the marinade, cover and leave for at least 20 minutes in the fridge, or for longer if you have the time.

When you are ready to cook, place the pork fillet on a baking tray lined with baking parchment and cook in the oven for 25–30 minutes. Every 5 minutes, brush the pork with the marinade that remains in the bottom of the bowl. When the pork is cooked, it should be golden on the outside and firm to the touch. Remove from the oven and sprinkle with half of the sesame seeds. Leave to rest and slice once cooled.

Cook the noodles following the packet instructions. Heat a wok or large frying pan and pour in the rapeseed oil. Add the sliced ginger and garlic, and cook for a 3–4 minutes, before adding in the greens. Add a couple of tablespoons of water to steam them and allow to cook for 3–4 minutes, stirring every now and then. While the greens are steaming, pour in any remaining marinade left over from the pork, as well as any pork juices that have come out as the pork has been resting.

Once the noodles are cooked, turn off the heat and drain. Toss them into the pan. Add the lime juice, soy sauce and a drizzle of sesame seed oil. Serve in bowls and top with a sprinkling of sesame seeds and the sliced pork.

CHICKEN, ROOT VEGETABLES AND ROSEMARY TRAY BAKE

Rich in protein, vitamins B12, B6 and C, potassium, iron and beta-carotene

Preparation time: 15 minutes
Cooking time: 35 minutes
Serves: 4

½ butternut squash, unpeeled, and cut into large chunks
4 parsnips, cut into chunks
8 baby new potatoes, halved
2 large red peppers, roughly chopped
2 large carrots, cut into large chunks
4 sprigs rosemary or thyme, chopped
2 tbsp good-quality runny honey
3 tbsp rapeseed oil
2 tbsp olive oil
4 large free-range chicken breasts, skin on, or 1 large chicken, jointed
    into 8 pieces (you can ask your butcher to do this)
sea salt and black pepper

Preheat the oven to fan 190°C/375°F/Gas 5. Place the chopped vegetables into a large baking dish, along with the rosemary or thyme, honey, both oils, and some salt and pepper. Toss the vegetables around so they become coated in all the oil and honey.

Rub the chicken with some salt and pepper and a little more oil, and put the pieces in the dish among the vegetables. Roast in the oven for 35 minutes or until the chicken is cooked through and the vegetables are tender. Serve immediately.

SLOW-COOKED LAMB WITH PRESERVED LEMONS

Zinc, vitamins C and B, and iron.

Preparation time: 20 minutes
Cooking time: 3 hours 30 minutes – 4 hours 30 minutes
Serves: 4–5

4 tbsp olive oil
650 g (1 lb 7 oz) lamb leg meat, cut into large cubes
2 tsp ground cumin
1 tsp ground coriander
1½ tsp paprika
1½ tsp chopped garlic
2 medium onions, sliced
6 medium-strength whole dried chillies
4 cloves
½ tsp ground cinnamon
550 ml (19 fl oz) tomato passata
50 g (2 oz) semi-dried tomatoes, or 40 g (1½ oz) sun-dried tomatoes
300 ml (½ pint) water
2 whole preserved lemons, or 12 wedges preserved lemons
large sprig mint, chopped
large sprig parsley, chopped
sea salt

To serve
rice or couscous

Preheat the oven to fan 160°C/325°F/Gas 3. You will need a robust 3 litre casserole dish with a snug-fitting lid, or use a frying pan and then a slow cooker. Add 1 tablespoon of olive oil to the casserole dish or frying pan, turn the heat up high and fry the chunks of lamb for about 5 minutes, until browned all over. Remove the lamb and set to one side.

Pour the remaining oil into the dish or pan, turn down the heat and gently fry the cumin, coriander, paprika and garlic for 3–4 minutes. Turn up the heat, throw in the onions and fry for 10–15 minutes until soft, stirring frequently.

Return the lamb to the dish or pan, turn down the heat along with the chillies, cloves, cinnamon, tomato passata, semi- or sun-dried tomatoes, water and preserved lemons. Bring to the boil, then turn down to a simmer.

Add half of the mint and parsley, and a little salt, then place the lid on the casserole dish and cook in the oven for 3–4 hours. Alternatively, transfer everything from the frying pan into a slow cooker and cook on high for 5–6 hours.

When ready to serve, garnish the stew with the remaining mint and parsley. Remove the chillies and the preserved lemon and throw away. Serve with rice or couscous.

SNACKS

FENNEL AND FLAXSEED OATCAKES

Rich in folate, magnesium, potassium, omega-3 and fibre

Preparation time: 20 minutes
Cooking time: 25 minutes
Makes: 16 oatcakes

225 g (8 oz) rolled oats
75 g (2½ oz) wholemeal flour, plus extra for rolling
2 tbsp ground flaxseed
1½ tsp fennel seeds, crushed or gently chopped
75 g (3 oz) salted butter, cold and cubed, plus extra for greasing
1 tsp bicarbonate of soda

85–100 ml (3–3½ fl oz) water from a recently boiled kettle

Preheat the oven to fan 180°C/350°F/Gas 4. In a large bowl, mix the oats with the flour, flaxseed and fennel seeds. Add the butter and, using your fingers, rub it into the mixture until it resembles breadcrumbs.

Add the bicarbonate of soda and gradually pour in the hot water. Mix until you have formed a dough. You may not need all the water.

Sprinkle the work surface generously with wholemeal flour and turn out the dough. Lightly knead it into a ball. Using a floured rolling pin, roll the dough out to 5 mm (¼ in) thick. Using a 5–6 cm (2–2½ in) cutter, cut out as many oatcakes as you can. Re-roll the excess and cut out the remaining dough.

Lightly oil or butter a non-stick baking tray and gently lift your oatcakes on to it. Bake them for around 25 minutes, until golden. Leave to cool completely on a wire rack before storing in an airtight container, ready for serving, snacking or spreading, as and when you wish.

PARMESAN SEEDED CRISPBREADS

Rich in vitamin B, fibre, folate, magnesium, potassium and iron

Preparation time: 10 minutes
Cooking time: 15–20 minutes
Makes: 12–14 crispbreads

225 g (8 oz) buckwheat flour
225 g (8 oz) wholemeal flour
75 g (2½ oz) sunflower seeds
75 g (2½ oz) pumpkin seeds
2 tbsp ground flaxseed

2 tbsp sesame seeds
75 g (2½ oz) pinhead or rolled oats
2 tbsp chia seeds
1 tsp salt
150 ml (5 fl oz) extra-virgin rapeseed or olive oil
240 ml (8½ fl oz) water
50 g (2 oz) Parmesan, finely grated
2 tbsp poppy seeds

Preheat the oven to fan 180°C/350°F/Gas 4. Cut 2 pieces of non-stick parchment paper to fit a large flat baking tray.

Mix all the dry ingredients in a bowl, make a well in the centre and add the oil and half of the water. Mix with your fingertips until you start to form a dough. Slowly add the remaining water until the dough is firm but not sticky. You may not need all of the water. Form the dough into a ball and place it on to the first layer of parchment. Place the second layer on top. Use the heel of your hand to flatten out the dough before using a rolling pin to roll it to the same size as your baking tray. It should be about 5 mm (¼ in) thick.

Lift your parchment containing the rolled dough and put it on to the baking tray. Remove the top layer of parchment and sprinkle over the Parmesan and poppy seeds. Bake in the oven for around 15–20 minutes, until golden brown and the bread has become crisp. Turn the tray around halfway through cooking to ensure it cooks evenly.

Once cooked, remove the tray from the oven and the parchment from underneath the crispbread. Using a large sharp knife or simply snap by hand for a more rustic effect – divide the crispbread into your desired shapes and sizes. I like random shapes: some big and some small. Leave to cool on a wire rack before storing in an airtight container or sandwich bags, ready to be eaten at your and your family's pleasure.

BEETROOT AND HAZELNUT DIP

Rich in folate, manganese, iron, omega-3 and 6, vitamin E and fibre

Preparation time: 10 minutes
Makes: 400 g (14 oz)

300 g (10½ oz) cooked un-pickled beetroot
100 g (3½ oz) toasted hazelnuts, skins on
zest of 1 large orange
1 tsp ground cumin
2 tbsp natural yoghurt
3 tbsp extra-virgin rapeseed, olive or flaxseed oil
sea salt and black pepper

To serve
crudités of your choice

Blitz all the ingredients except the salt and papper in a large blender or food processor until smooth. Season to taste and serve, or keep in an airtight container. This dip will last for 2–3 days in the fridge. Serve with crudités such as sliced peppers, cucumber and celery.

Tip: It's a good idea to make a batch of some sort of dip every couple of days, especially in the third trimester and during breastfeeding when you may feel like snacking more.

CREAMY SPINACH DIP

Rich in iron, folate, magnesium, calcium and vitamin C

Preparation time: 10 minutes
Makes: 400 g (14 oz)

2 tsp olive oil
2 shallots, chopped

1 small onion, diced, or 4 sspring onions, sliced
1 tbsp crushed garlic
225 g (8 oz) spinach or kale leaves
2 tsp lemon juice
100 g (3½ oz) goat's/sheep's/organic cow's yoghurt
50 g (2 oz) crumbled feta
2 tbsp chopped dill
¼ tsp salt (only if needed)
freshly ground black pepper

Heat the oil in a wok or large sauté pan over a medium heat. Cook
the shallots and onion for 3–4 minutes, then add the garlic and sauté
for another minute. Add the spinach or kale and cook until wilted
(kale needs to be cooked for a few more minutes than spinach, until
it softens). Scoop the mixture into a food processor and pulse until
almost puréed. Add the remaining ingredients and pulse once only.
Add black pepper to taste.

APPLE CHIPS

Rich in fibre and vitamin C

Preparation time: 15 minutes
Cooking time: 30 minutes
Makes: 4 servings

4 apples
4 tbsp good-quality runny honey
2 tsp ground cinnamon

Preheat the oven to fan 160°C/325°F/Gas 3. Line 2–3 baking sheets
with non-stick parchment paper. Slice the apples as thinly as you
can, preferably around 2 mm thick, either using a mandolin or a
sharp knife. Leave the skin on but remove any pips.

Lay the apple slices on to the lined baking sheets, making sure
they are not touching.

Heat the honey and cinnamon in a small saucepan until melted. Brush each apple with a little of the mixture and bake in the oven for 15 minutes. Remove the trays from the oven, turn over each slice and brush them again with the remaining mixture. Bake in the oven for a further 15 minutes. Once the apple slices are crisp and slightly golden and firm to the touch, remove them from the oven and leave to cool on a wire rack.

Once cooled they can be stored in an airtight container for 4–5 days, ready for snacking.

Tip: You may want to swap the trays over – top shelf to bottom shelf, and bottom shelf to top shelf – to ensure even cooking.

5-MINUTE MACKEREL PÂTÉ

Rich in protein, DHA, EPA, iodine, vitamin A, vitamin D, and vitamin B

Preparation time: 5 minutes
Serves: 2

200 g (7 oz) smoked mackerel
2 tbsp cottage cheese
1 tbsp half-fat crème fraîche
juice of 1 lemon
horseradish to taste
freshsly ground black pepper to taste

Put all the ingredients into a food processor and pulse until combined and to the texture you prefer.

Tips:

- Serve with a salad and baked sweet potato for lunch or supper, or dip into it with oatcakes (see page 199), rice cakes or spelt crackers for a perfect snack.

- You can substitute the mackerel for trout, tuna or salmon if you prefer.

TOFU-NUT BALLS

Rich in protein, fibre, vitamin B and magnesium

Preparation time: 10 minutes
Cooking time: 1 hour 15 minutes
Makes: approximately 20 balls

olive or sesame oil
90 g (3¼ oz) short grain brown rice
240 ml (8½ fl oz) water
2 tbsp tamari (wheat-free soy sauce)
225 g (8 oz) soft tofu, mashed
60 g (2 oz) ground almonds
25 g (1 oz) finely ground fresh breadcrumbs, or 75 g (3 oz) shop-
*   bought dried breadcrumbs*
sea salt

Preheat the oven to fan 180°C/350°F/Gas 4 and lightly oil a baking sheet. Place the rice and water into a small saucepan. Bring to the boil, cover, and lower the heat to the gentlest possible simmer. Cook until the rice is very soft; about 35–45 minutes.

Put the tamari and half of the mashed tofu into a blender or food processor, and add about three quarters of the cooked rice. Blend to a thick paste. Place the remaining tofu into a medium-size bowl. Add the blended mixture, along with the almonds, breadcrumbs, and remaining rice. Season to taste. Using your hands, form the batter into 2½ cm (1 in) balls. Put them on to the baking tray and cook in the oven for 30 minutes. Serve hot as a snack or with a green salad for lunch.

Tip: If you prefer, you can sauté the balls in a little oil in a frying pan for about 15 minutes instead.

CHICKEN STOCK OR BROTH

Rich in protein, minerals and amino acids

Preparation time: 10 minutes
Cooking time: at least 6 hours
Makes: 1–1.5 litres

chicken carcass, flesh removed
1 bay leaf
capful of apple cider vinegar, or juice of 1 lemon
1 onion (unpeeled)
1 celery stick (leaves and stalk)
1 carrot (unpeeled)
fresh or dried herbs of your choice, such as sage and rosemary

Put all the ingredients into a large stock pot or casserole dish. Add enough water to cover the carcass. Cover with a lid and bring to the boil over a high heat. Reduce the heat to low and simmer for at least 6 hours. The longer the stock is left to slowly cook, the greater the nutrient content. I cook mine on a low heat in my slow cooker for 12 hours to maximise the nutrient content. Strain the broth into a large bowl or jug through a fine sieve; discard the bones, vegetables and herbs.

Tips:
- You can make lamb or beef stock in the same way. Simply replace the chicken carcass with lamb or beef bones.
- You can roast a whole chicken and use the cooked meat for snacks or to add into soups, then use the carcass to make stock.

SAUERKRAUT

Rich in probiotics and vitamin K

Preparation time: At least 3 days

1 medium cabbage, finely shredded
1 tbsp caraway seeds
1 tbsp sea salt

Mix all the ingredients together in a bowl. Transfer to a sterilised 500 ml (17½ fl oz) Mason jar (or other jar with a lid), adding some pressure so that the cabbage is tightly packed. This should leave at least a 2½ cm (1 in) gap between the top of the cabbage and the lid of the jar so the mixture can 'grow' during the fermentation process. Put on the lid tightly and store in a dark cupboard at room temperature for 3 days. After 3 days, transfer to the fridge.

Add a dessertspoon to salads, or eat as a snack with cheese and Fennel and Flaxseed Oatcakes (see page 200).

Tips:
- You can use any type of cabbage or, even better, a mix of varieties.
- Sauerkraut improves with age so you can leave it in your fridge for at least 1 month.

KEFIR

Rich in vitamin K, vitamin B, prebiotics and probiotics

Preparation time: 5 minutes
Makes: 900 ml (1½ pints)

1 tbsp kefir grains
900 ml (1½ pints) organic whole milk

Put the kefir grains and milk into a large glass jar. Cover tightly. Leave out at room temperature, but not in direct sunlight, for 12–24 hours. It will be ready sooner in warm weather than in cold weather. Shake the kefir gently a couple of times if you remember.

When the kefir is ready, you will see kefir grains coagulate at the top of the jar. Spoon off these grains and them put into a separate container for your next batch. You can also strain the grains out by using a small sieve or colander. Kefir will last 3–4 weeks in the fridge.

Tips
- You can buy kefir grains at many health food stores or online.
- You can use cow's, goat's, coconut, yak or other types of milk. They can be skimmed, semi-skimmed or whole milk (preferable).
- For someone who is extremely sensitive, you can even make kefir from water. Use 950 ml (33½ fl oz) of water, 60 g (2 oz) of organic brown sugar, 1 tsp of molasses and 50 g (1.8 oz) of kefir grains.

SWEET TREATS

BLUEBERRY ICE CREAM

Rich in magnesium, zinc, vitamin C and antioxidants

Preparation time: 10 minutes
Freezing time: approximately 2-3 hours
Serves: 2

100 g (3½ oz) raw cashews
175 g (6 oz) frozen blueberries
85 ml (3 fl oz) water
2 tbsp agave syrup

Whizz all the ingredients in a blender until smooth. Transfer the mixture to an ice cream maker and freeze according to the manufacturer's instructions. Once frozen (usually 2–3 hours), transfer the ice cream to a freezer-proof container, cover and freeze until firm.

If you don't have an ice cream maker, transfer the mixture to a shallow freezer-proof dish and place in the freezer until it just starts to harden around the edges. Whisk vigorously with a fork to break up the ice crystals and then refreeze until firm.

NOURISH BAR

Rich in iron, vitamin B, calcium and magnesium

Preparation time: 50 minutes
Cooking time: 1 hour 30 minutes
Makes: 12

250 g (9 oz) rice flour
125 g (4 oz) rolled oats
50 g (2 oz) ground almonds
50 g (2 oz) linseeds
50 g (2 oz) sesame seeds
125 g (4½ oz) organic dried apricots, chopped
200 g (7 oz) organic cranberry and raisin mix
1 tsp mixed spice
3 pieces crystallised ginger, finely chopped
50 g (2 oz) sunflower seeds
3 tbsp apple juice
600 ml (1 pint) almond or organic whole milk
1 tbsp malt extract
25 g (1 oz) flaked almonds

To serve
nut butter

Preheat the oven to fan 190°C/375°F/Gas 5. Grease and line a 900 g (2 lb) loaf tin. Put all the dry ingredients except for the flaked almonds into a bowl and stir. Pour in the apple juice, milk and malt extract, and mix together. Set aside for 45 minutes. Pour the mixture into the tin and level with a spoon. Scatter over the almonds, cover with foil and bake for 25 minutes. Remove the foil and cook for a further 20 minutes until a skewer comes out clean. Allow to cool slightly in the tin first then transfer to a wire rack. Slice and serve with nut butter.

Tip: If the listed dried fruits don't take your fancy, replace with those that do – keep to the same measurements. The bars can be frozen for up to 3 months.

DRINKS

GREEN GOODNESS SMOOTHIE

Rich in folate, vitamin C, magnesium, vitamin E, anthocyanins

Preparation time: 5 minutes
Makes: approximately 600 ml (1 pint)

1 scoop (or according to packet instructions) of protein powder such as
     hemp or rice
½ avocado
1 tsp coconut butter
2 tbsp blueberries, blackberries or raspberries (fresh or frozen)
handful of leafy greens of your choice
freshly ground cinnamon or vanilla powder to taste
almond milk

Put all the ingredients except for the almond milk into a blender. Add enough almond milk to just cover the ingredients blend until smooth.

Tips:
- Drink for a great start to the day or as a snack.
- If you need it to be a little sweeter, add 1 dessertspoon of agave syrup or manuka honey.

DEEPLY NOURISHING SPICE TEA

Rich in vitamin C and gingerols

Preparation time: 10 minutes
Makes: 600 ml (1 pint)

good-quality honey to taste (optional)
1 tbsp grated ginger
½ lemongrass, chopped
juice of 1 lemon, or 1 tbsp apple cider vinegar
½ tsp turmeric
½ tsp cayenne pepper

Put all of the ingredients into a large teapot. If you are using honey, stir well to make a paste. Add 600 ml (1 pint) of boiling water and leave to steep for 5 minutes (or longer). Using a tea strainer, pour into a mug.

Tip: In my early weeks of pregnancy when I was experiencing a bit of nausea I made this at the start of every day, keeping the ingredients in the pot and adding water throughout the day.

FORTIFYING MAMA TEA

Rich in vitamins C, B, K and A

Preparation time: 5
Serves: 4–5

1 tsp dried nettle leaves
1 tsp dried raspberry leaves

1 tsp dried dandelion leaves
1 tsp grated cinnamon
pinch of grated nutmeg
1–2 cloves

Combine the ingredients together in a Mason jar or other airtight container. Mix well, cover wiwth the lid and store. When making the tea, add 1 teaspoon of the dried mixture per person into a teapot. Pour in boiling water and leave to steep for 5 minutes. Using a tea strainer, pour into a mug.

Note: I had the idea for this this tea with inspiration from Susun Weed, a woman of great herbal wisdom and a mother herself.

Tips:
- Continue to add hot water to the teapot throughout the day.
- Add honey for a bit of sweetness if you need it. If you are breast-feeding and your baby is a little windy, you can add a teaspoon of fennel seeds or a cardamom pod into this mixture too.

RESOURCES

Henrietta Norton Nutrition Clinic
www.henriettanorton.com
email: clinic@henriettanorton.com
020 7235 8900 (extension 2)
Clinics in London and Sussex

PREGNANCY SUPPORT

Miscarriage Association
www.miscarriageassociation.org.uk

National Childbirth Trust
www.nct.org.uk
0300 330 0700

NHS nutritional advice
www.nhs.uk/conditions/pregnancy-and-baby/pages/healthy-pregnancy-diet.aspx

PNI
Support for postnatal depression
www.pni.org.uk

TAMBA (Twins & Multiple Births Association)
www.tamba.org.uk
0800 138 0509

Tommy's
www.tommys.org
0800 0147 800

ENVIRONMENTAL HEALTH

Drinkaware
www.drinkaware.co.uk
020 7766 9900

Environmental Working Group
www.ewg.org

Foods Standards Agency (FSA)
www.food.gov.uk

Foresight preconceptual care.
www.foresight-preconception.org.uk
01275 878953
info@foresight-preconception.org.uk

Marine Conservation Society (MCS UK)
www.mcsuk.org

NHS advice on stopping smoking
www.nhs.uk/smokefree

QUIT smoking support
www.quit.org.uk
0800 002 200

Women's Environmental Network
www.wen.org.uk
020 7481 9004

HEALTH STORES

Goodness Direct
www.goodnessdirect.co.uk

Infinity Foods
www.infinityfoods.co.uk

Natures Healthbox
www.natureshealthbox.co.uk

Planet Organic
www.planetorganic.com

Wholefoods Market
www.wholefoodsmarket.com

ORGANIC VEGETABLE AND MEAT DELIVERY

Abel & Cole
www.abelandcole.co.uk

Find Local Produce
www.findlocalproduce.co.uk

Riverford
www.riverford.co.uk

If you live outside of a city, check your area for local delivery schemes.

SUPPLEMENTS

Herb Hands Healing
www.herbs-hands-healing.co.uk
01379 608 201

Wild Nutrition
www.wildnutrition.com
01273 906 410

HERBALISTS

Michael McIntyre
www.michael-mcintyre.com
01993 830 419

National Institute of Medical Herbalists
www.nimh.org.uk
01392 426 022

NUTRITIONAL THERAPISTS

**British Association for Applied Nutrition and Nutritional
Therapy (BANT)**
www.bant.org.uk
theadministrator@bant.org.uk
0870 606 1284

MEDITATION

British Meditation Society
www.britishmeditationsociety.org

HeadSpace
www.headspace.com

HOMEOPATHY

British Homeopathic Association
www.britishhomeopathic.org
01582 408 675

Helios
www.helios.co.uk
01892 536 393

Lisa Bullen
www.lisabullenhomeopathy.co.uk

Society of Homeopaths
www.homeopathy-soh.org

ACUPUNCTURE

Anna de Moore
www.annademoor.co.uk

The British Acupuncture Council
www.acupuncture.org.uk
020 8735 0400

Emma Cannon
www.emmacannon.co.uk

Rick Mudie
www.sussexacupuncture.co.uk

HYPNOBIRTHING

Hypnobirthing: The Mongan Method
www.hypnobirthing.co.uk

CRANIAL OSTEOPATHY

College of Cranio-Sacral Therapy
www.ccst.co.uk
020 7483 0120

Institute of Osteopathy
www.osteopathy.org

YOGA

British Wheel of Yoga
www.bwy.org.uk
01529 306 851

Michelle Pearce, yoga teacher & massage
michellecpearce@live.co.uk

YogaGlo Online yoga classes
www.yogaglo.com

PILATES

Pilates Foundation
www.pilatesfoundation.com

ANTENATAL CLASSES

Lulubaby
www.lulubaby.co.uk
020 7736 6665

National Childbirth Trust
www.nct.org.uk
0300 330 0700

Prenatal Classroom
www.theprenatalclassroom.com
07940 589 021

BREASTFEEDING SUPPORT

Association of Breastfeeding Mothers
www.abm.me.uk
0300 330 5453

Breastfeeding Network
www.breastfeedingnetwork.org.uk
0300 100 0212

La Leche League
www.laleche.org.uk
0845 120 2918

RECOMMENDED COOKERY BOOKS

- *A Modern Way to Eat* by Anna Jones
- *Deliciously Ella* by Ella Woodward
- *Plenish: Juices to Boost, Cleanse & Heal* by Kara Rosen

- *The Natural Cook: Eating the Seasons from Root to Fruit* by Tom Hunt
- *The Art of Eating Well* by Hemsley & Hemsley

FURTHER READING

- *Healthy Beauty* by Samuel S. Epstein, M.D. (BenBella Books, 2011)
- *Homeopathy for Mother and Baby: Pregnancy, Birth & The Postnatal Year* by Miranda Castro (Homoeopathic Supply Company, 2005)
- *The Nourishing Traditions Book of Baby & Child Care* by Sally Fallon Morell (New Trends Publishing Inc, 2013)
- *Wise Woman Herbal for the Childbearing Year* by Susun Weed (New Leaf Distribution Company, 1986)

REFERENCES

CHAPTER 2

Barker, D. (1998) *Mothers Babies and Health in Later Life*, 2nd ed. Edinburgh: Churchill Livingstone, pp.134–135

Earth Summit Report (1991)

Gaydos, L.J. et al. (2014) 'H3K27me and PRC2 transmit a memory of repression across generations and during development', *Science*, 345 (6203): 1515–1518

Jacka, F.N. et al. (2013) 'Maternal and early postnatal nutrition and mental health of offspring by age 5 years: a prospective cohort study', *Journal of American Academy of Child & Adolescence Psychiatry*, 52 (10): 1038–47

Mason, J.B. et al. (2014) 'The first 500 days of life: policies to support maternal nutrition', *Global Health Action*, 7 '23623'

Mayer, A.M. (1997) 'Historical changes in the mineral content of fruits and vegetables', *British Food Journal*, 99 (6): 207–211

McArdle, Prof. J.H. et al. (2013) 'Introduction to early life and later disease', British Nutrition Foundation (eds) *Nutrition and Development: Short and Long Term Consequences for Health*, Chichester, West Sussex: Wiley-Blackwell, pp.238–239

Office for National Statistics and Health and Social Care Information Centre

Roseboom et al. (2006) 'The Dutch Famine and its long-term consequences for adult health', *Early Human Development*, 82: 485–91

CHAPTER 4

Brenna, J.T. et al. (2014) 'Docosahexaenoic acid and human brain develop-ment: Evidence that a dietary supply is needed for optimal development', *Journal of Human Evolution*, Dec, 77: 99–106

Simopoulos, A.P. (2003) 'Important of the ratio of omega-6/omega-3 essential fatty acids: Evolutionary aspects', *World Review of Nutrition and Dietetics*, 92: 1–22

Ryan, A.S. et al. (2010) 'Effects of long-chain polyunsaturated fatty acid supplementation on neurodevelopment in childhood: a review of human studies', *Prostaglandins Leukotriene Essential Fatty Acids*, 82 (4–6): 305–14

CHAPTER 5

Hodgetts, V. et al. (2014) 'Effectiveness of folic acid supplementation in pregnancy on reducing the risk of small-for-gestational age neonates: A population study, systemative review and meta-analysis', *International Journal of Obstetrics and Gynaecology*, Nov, 26, doi: 10.1111/1471-0528.13202. [Epub ahead of print]

Jiang, X. et al. (2012) 'Maternal choline intake alters the epigenetic state of fetal cortisol-regulating genes in humans', *FASEB Journal*, Aug, 26 (8): 3563–74

McArdle, Prof. J.H. et al. (2013) 'Introduction to Early Life and Later Disease', British Nutrition Foundation (eds) *Nutrition and Development: Short and Long Term Consequences for Health*, Chichester, West Sussex: Wiley-Blackwell: pp.238–239

Miyake (2015) 'Dietary vitamin D intake and prevalence of depressive symptoms during pregnancy in Japan', *Nutrition*, 31 (1): 160–5, doi: 10.1016/j.nut.2014.06.013 [Epub 2014 Jul 19]

SACN (2011)

Schnoenaker, D. (2014) 'The association between dietary factors and gestational hypertension and pre-eclampsia: A systematic review and meta-analysis of observational studies', *BioMed Central*, Sep, 22, 12(1): 157 [Epub ahead of print]

Singla, R. et al. (2014) 'Relationship between preeclampsia and vitamin D deficiency: A case control study', *Archives of Gynecology & Obstetrics*, doi: 10.1007/s00404-014-3550-8 [Epub ahead of print]

Stelmach (2014) 'Cord serum 25-hydroxyvitamin D correlates with early childhood viral-induced wheezing', *Respiratory Medicine*, Nov, 3, pii: S0954-6111(14)00366-7. doi: 10.1016/j.rmed.2014. 10.016 [Epub ahead of print]

CHAPTER 6

Al-Saleh et al. (2014) 'Birth outcome measures and maternal exposure to heavy metals (lead, cadmium and mercury) in Saudi Arabian population. *International Journal of Hygeine and Environmental Health*, Mar, 217 (2–3): 205–18

Ashley-Martin, J. et al. (2014) 'A birth cohort study to investigate the association between prenatal phthalate and bisphenol A exposures and fetal markers of metabolic dysfunction', *Environmental Health*, Oct, 22: 13–84

Daley, C.A. et al. (2010) 'A review of fatty acid profiles and antioxidant content in grass-fed and grain-fed beef', *Nutrition Journal*, 9: (10), doi:10.1186/1475-2891-9-10

Leheska, J.M. et al. (2008) 'Effects of conventional and grass-feeding systems on the nutrient composition of beef', *Journal of Animal Sciences*, Dec, 86 (12): 3575–85, doi: 10.2527/jas.2007-0565

Leventakou, V. (2014) 'Fish intake during pregnancy, fetal growth and gestational length in 19 European birth cohort studies', *American Journal of Clinical Nutrition*, Mar, 99 (3): 506–16, doi: 10.3945/ajcn.113.067421 [Epub 2013 Dec 11]

Ponnampalam, E.N. et al. (2006) 'Effect of feeding systems on omega-3 fatty acids, conjugated linoleic acid and trans fatty acids in Australian beef cuts: potential impact on human health', *Asian Pacific Journal of Clinical Nutrition*, 15 (1): 21–9

Suez, J. et al. (2014), 'Artificial sweeteners induce glucose intolerance by altering the gut microbiota', *Nature*, Oct, 514: 181–186

CHAPTER 7

Bizzaro, G. (2014) 'Vitamin D and autoimmune thyroid diseases: Facts and unresolved questions', *Immunological Research*, Nov, 19 [Epub ahead of print]

Miles et al. (2014) 'Maternal diet and its influence on the development of allergic disease', *Clinical & Experimental Allergy*, Nov, 14, doi: 10.1111/cea.12453 [Epub ahead of print]

Munyaka. P.M. et al. (2014) 'External influence of early childhood establishment of gut microbiota and subsequent health implications', *Front Pediatrics*, Oct, 2 (109)

Oberlander, T.F. (2008) 'Prenatal exposure to maternal depression, neonatal methylation of human glucocorticoid receptor gene (NR3CI) and infant cortisol stress responses', *Epigenetics*, Mar–Apr, 3 (2): 97–106

Schmidt et al. (2014) 'Maternal intake of supplemental iron and risk of autism spectrum disorder, *American Journal of Epidemiology*, Nov, 1, 180 (9): 890–900

Vanderlelie, J. (2014) 'First trimester multivitamin/mineral use is associated with reduced risk of pre-eclampsia among overweight and obese women', *Maternal and Child Nutrition*, May, 22, doi: 10.1111/mcn.12133

Vinson, J.A. and Bose, P. (1998) 'Comparative bioavailability to humans of ascorbic acid alone or in a citrus extract', *American Journal of Clinical Nutrition*, Sep, 48 (3): 601–4

CHAPTER 10

Freeman, M.P. et al. (2006) 'Omega-3 fatty acids: Evidence basis for treatment and future research in psychiatry', *Journal of Clinical Psychiatry*, 67, 1954–67

Hibbeln, J.R. (2002) 'Seafood consumption, the DHA content of mothers' milk and prevalence rates of postpartum depression: A cross-national, ecological analysis', *Journal of Affective Disorders*, 69: 15–29

Munyaka, P.M. et al. (2014) 'External influence of early childhood establishment of gut microbiota and subsequent health implications', *Front Pediatrics*, Oct, 2 (109)

Numakawa, T. et al. (2014) 'The role of brain-derived neurotrophic factor in comorbid depression: possible linkage with steroid hormones, cytokines, and nutrition', *Front Psychiatry*, Sep, 26(5) 136, doi: 10.3389/fpsyt.2014.00136

Rees, A.M. et al. (2005) 'Role of omega-3 fatty acids as a treatment for depression in the perinatal period', *Australia & New Zealand Journal of Psychiatry*, 39: 274–80

CHAPTER 12

Chau et al. (2015) 'Probiotics for infantile colic: a randomized, double-blind, placebo-controlled trial investigating lactobacillus reuteri DSM 17938. *Journal of Pediatrics*, Jan, 166, (1): 74–78

Kianifar, H. et al. (2014) 'Synbiotic in the management of infantile colic: a randomised controlled trial', *Journal of Paediatric Child Health*, Oct, 50 (10): 801–5

Kramer, M.S. et al. (2001) 'Promotion of breastfeeding intervention trial (PROBIT): A randomized trial in the Republic of Belarus', *Journal of the American Medical Association*, Jan, 24–31, 285(4): 413–20

Savino, F. et al. (2010) 'Lactobacillus reuteri DSM 17938 in infantile colic: A randomized, double-blind, placebo-controlled trial', *Pediatrics*, Sep, 126 (3): e526–33

Teter, B.B. et al. (1990) 'Milk fat in depression in C57B1/6J mice consuming partially hydrogenated fats', *Journal of Nutrition*, 120: 818–824

Thompson, A.L. et al. (2012) 'Developmental origins of obesity: Early feeding environments, infant growth, and the intestinal microbiome', *American Journal of Human Biology*, May–Jun, 24 (3): 350–60, doi: 10.1002/ajhb.22254

Walker, W.A. et al. (2015) 'Breast milk, microbiota, and intestinal immune homeostasis', *Pediatric Research*, Jan, 77 (1–2): 220–228, doi: 10.1038/pr.2014.160 [Epub 2014 Oct 13]

INDEX

ACKNOWLEDGEMENTS

As with the journey to pregnancy, the process of writing a book is never the result of one person alone. It would have been impossible, let alone enjoyable, without the love and support of my precious family. Their endless 'cheerleading' gave me unwavering support throughout the whole process from conception to fruition. Being pregnant during the writing of this book with our third beautiful boy has made this that much more special too.

An enormous thank you to Sam Jackson for asking me to write the book – something I have always wanted to do, and for Michelle Porter and Dawn Bates for their eagle eye for detail. Indeed to all the team at Ebury, thank you for your structure and support throughout.

I am so grateful, too, for the delicious recipe contributions from chef Sophie Wright and the wisdom of yoga teacher Michelle Pearce, both of whom nourished and stretched me throughout my pregnancy and the writing of this book.

But mostly, my gratitude is for the women with whom I have had the gift of working with during their journey from conception to birth. It has and continues to be a deeply inspiring, humbling and learning experience that I hope will never stop. Thank you to you all

'Women are the carriers of life. We hold the fruit of our loving beneath our hearts. For too long we have lost touch with the fullness of this mystery due to modern, technological culture.... now is the time to be fully who we are throughout the childbearing years – guardians and nurturers of new life.'

Susun Weed, *Wise Woman Herbal*